MANUAL

OF

VETERINARY SPECIFIC

HOMEOPATHY...

MANUAL
OF
VETERINARY SPECIFIC
HOMEOPATHY,

COMPRISING DISEASES OF

HORSES, CATTLE, SHEEP, HOGS, DOGS AND POULTRY,

AND THEIR

SPECIFIC HOMEOPATHIC TREATMENT.

BY

F.HUMPHREYS

GYAN

Published by

Gyan Publishing House
5, Ansari Road
Daryaganj, New Delhi-110002
Phone: 011-47034999, 9811692060
E-mail: books@gyanbooks.com

Distribution Network
gyanbooks.com
India, USA, Canada, UK, Australia

ISBN: 978-93-6280-141-8 (HB)
First Published, 1882

2nd Impression 2024

Printed at: Gyan Press, Delhi.

MANUAL OF VETERINARY SPECIFIC HOMEOPATHY ..
Author: F.HUMPHREYS

MANUAL

OF

VETERINARY SPECIFIC HOMEOPATHY,

COMPRISING DISEASES OF

Horses, Cattle, Sheep, Hogs, Dogs and Poultry,

AND THEIR

SPECIFIC HOMEOPATHIC TREATMENT.

THIRD REVISED AND ENLARGED EDITION.

BY

F. HUMPHREYS, M. D.,

LATE PROFESSOR, AUTHOR, Etc., Etc.

HUMPHREYS' SPECIFIC HOMEOPATHIC MEDICINE CO.,

General Depot:

109 FULTON STREET, NEW YORK.

Retail Depot:

862 BROADWAY, just above 17th Street.

1882.

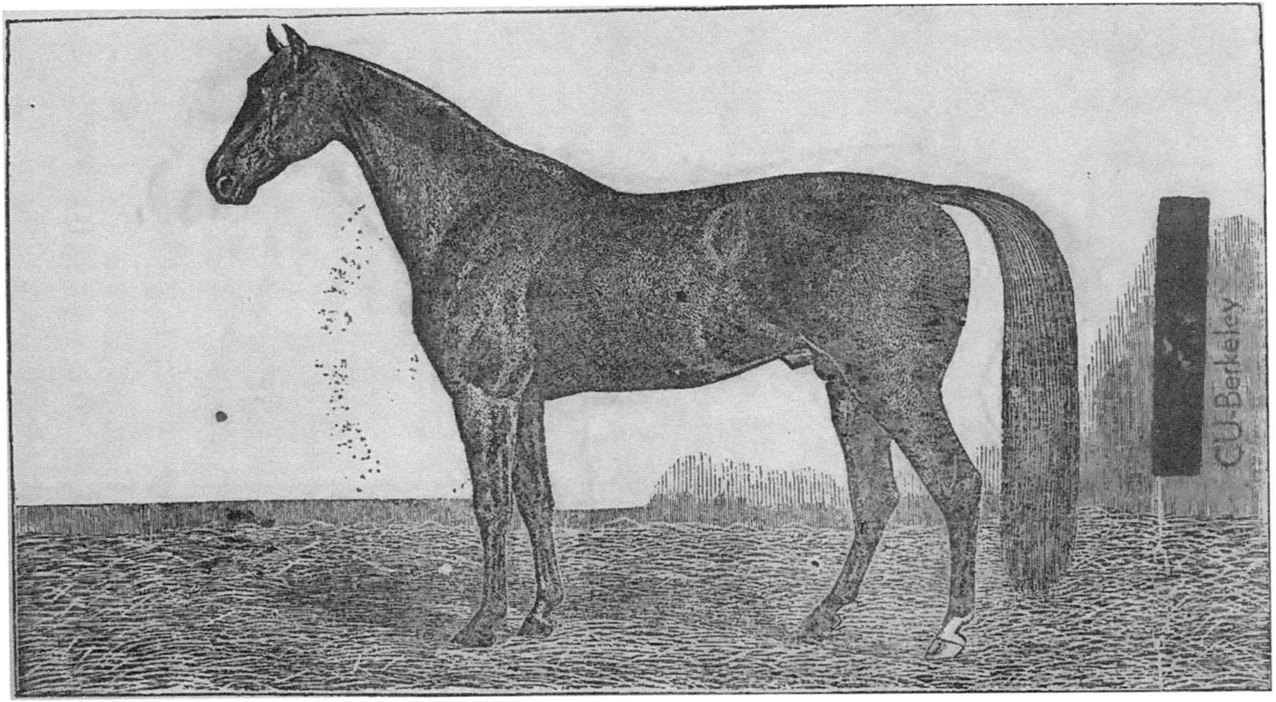

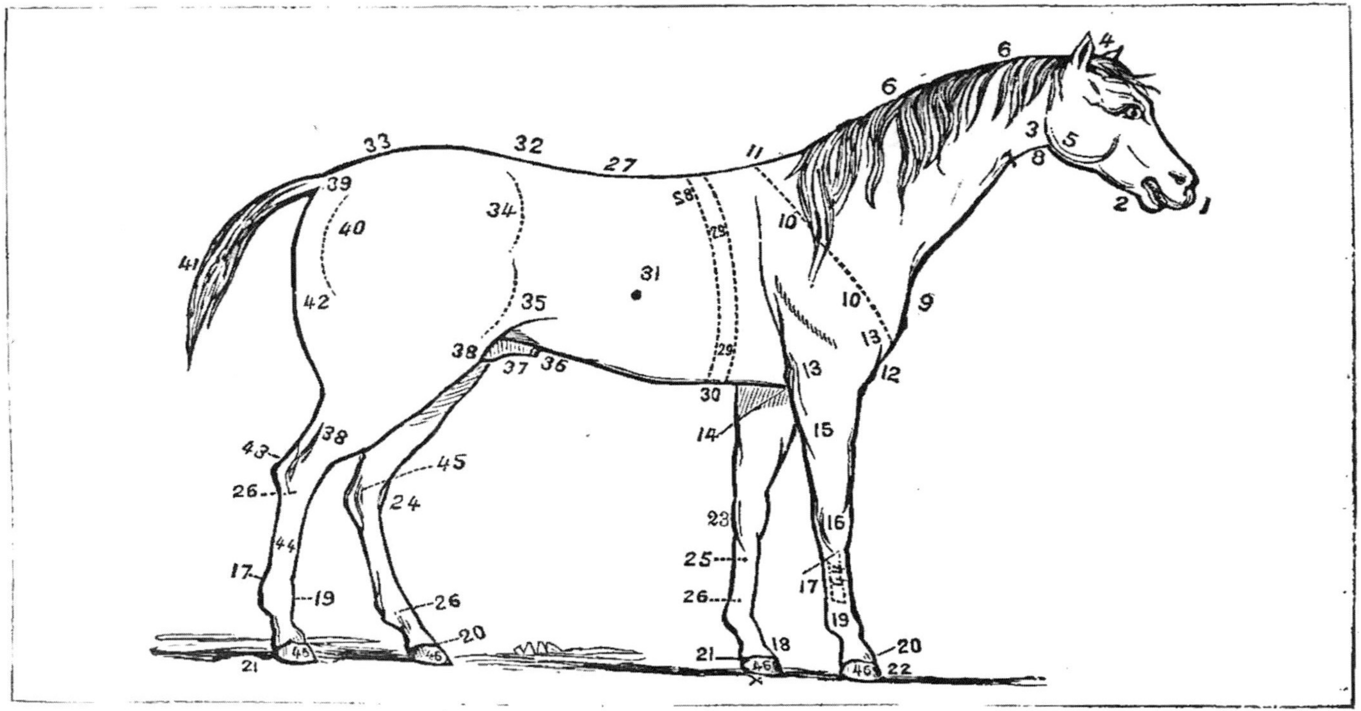
1
2
3
4
5
6
6
8
9
10
10
11
12
13
13
14
15
16
17
17
18
19
19
20
20
21
21
22
23
24
25
26
26
26
27
28
29
29
30
31
32
33
34
35
36
37
38
38
39
40
41
42
43
44
45
46
46
46
46

SKETCH OF A HORSE,

Showing the principal points and the external parts to be examined for injuries, defects and diseases.

1. Muzzle.
2. Place of Fistula from Teeth.
3. Place of Mumps.
4. Place of Poll-evil.
5. Angle of Jaw.
6, 6. Crest.
7. Place of Fistula from Vein.
8. Throttle, Thropple or Wind-pipe.
9. Shoulder-point: place of Sores from Harness.
10, 10. Shoulder-blade.
11. Withers; sometimes the seat of Fistula: height of horses reckoned from the Ground to the Withers.
12. Front of Chest, Bosom, or Breast.
13, 13. The True Arm. (See Skeleton.)
14. Elbow: often the seat of Tumours.
15. Arm, or Fore-arm.
16. Knee, or Wrist; may be swelled, having a fungous growth; or the skin may have been broken—evidence of a fall.*
17, 17. Back Sinew: place of Curb.
18. Place of Disease of Skin above the Coronet—Crown scab.
19, 19. Fetlock, or Pastern Joint
20. Coronet.
21, 21. Heel.
22. Contracted Hoof.
23. Mallenders.
24. Sallenders.
25. Seat of Splint, or Exostosis, on Side of Cannon-bone.
26, 26, 26. Seat of Bursal Enlargements.
27. Back, or spine.
28. Place of Saddle-galls.
29, 29. Girth, or Circumference in Measurement.
30. Place of Injury from Pressure of Girth.
31. Barrel, or Middle-piece,
32. Loins.
33. Croup.
34. Haunch.
35. Flank.
36. Seat of Warts.
37. Sheath, or Prepuce.
38, 38. Gas-skin, or Lower Thigh
39. Root of the Dock, or Tail.
40. Hip-joint—Round or Whirl-bone.
41. Rat-tail.
42. The Quarters.
43. Point of the Hock; seat of Capped-hock.
44. 44. Cannon-bone.
45. Place of Spavin.
46, 46. Hoof.

SKELETON

OF THE

HORSE.

SHOWING THE PRINCIPAL BONES AND REGIONS.

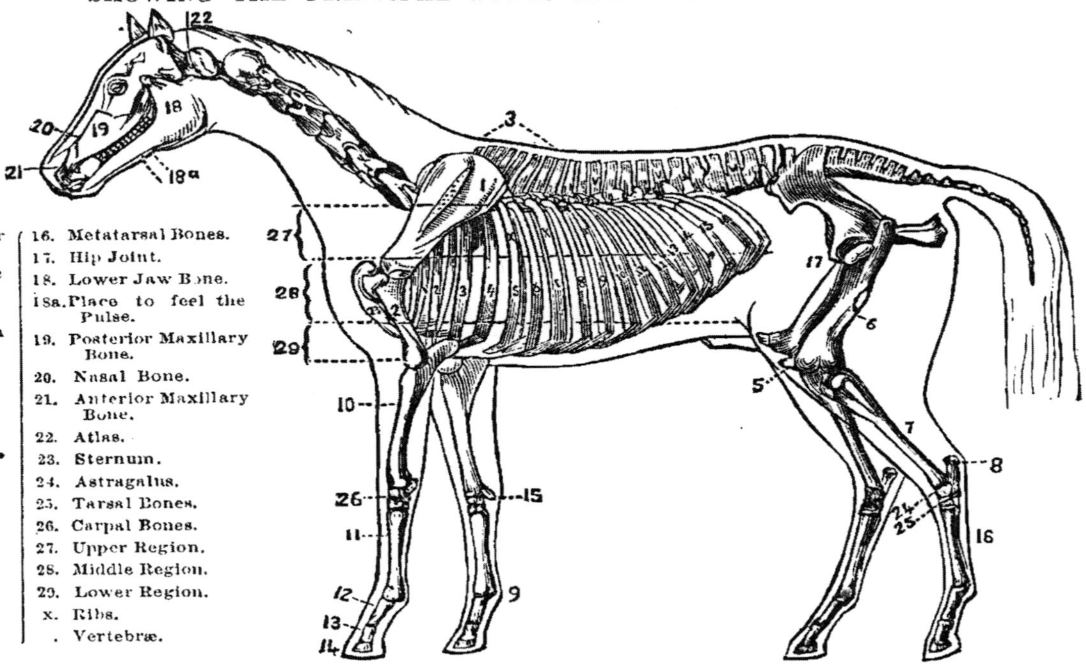

1. Scapula, or Shoulder Blade.
2. Humerus, or True Arm.
3. Withers.
4. Pelvis, or Haunch Bone.
5. Patella, or Stifle.
6. Femur.
7. Tibia.
8. Os Calcis.
9. Sesamoid Bones.
10. Radius.
11. Metacarpal Bones.
12. Great, or Upper, Pastern bone.
13. Small, or Lower, Pastern Bone.
14. Os Pedis.
15. Trapezium.
16. Metatarsal Bones.
17. Hip Joint.
18. Lower Jaw Bone.
18a. Place to feel the Pulse.
19. Posterior Maxillary Bone.
20. Nasal Bone.
21. Anterior Maxillary Bone.
22. Atlas.
23. Sternum.
24. Astragalus.
25. Tarsal Bones.
26. Carpal Bones.
27. Upper Region.
28. Middle Region.
29. Lower Region.

x. Ribs.

. Vertebræ.

PREFACE.

THE world owes much to Homœopathy—more, probably, than has ever been told, or will ever be known. It is something to be emancipated from drugs, from lancets, leeches, blisters and poisons; but it is more, to be relieved from the fear of them, and to be restored and preserved by forces mild as love, and gentle as the dews of heaven—forces unknown and unrevealed, until elicited by the genius of this system.

But these benefits are not confined to the human species. Animals may enjoy them as well; and heaven knows how much they need them. For to them the day of sickness is not merely the day of doom, but of suffering and of torture as well. Ignorance and cruelty seem to have controlled this branch of medicine—not that men are of necessity careless in regard to the lives of their animals, or designed cruel as to the measures used to restore them when sick; but so little real knowledge prevails concerning their diseases, and so much error as to the proper methods of cure, that the most absurd and cruel measures almost of necessity prevail with corresponding results. Some judicious stock-owners, taught by experience the fatality of the common methods of treatment, notwithstanding the torture and expense, have more humanely, if not more wisely, abandoned all treatment, preferring to let nature contend with disease alone, rather than with disease and drugs united. But, thanks to Homœopathy, there is a better way.

For many years past, Homœopathy has been applied to the diseases of all domestic animals in Europe, with the most brilliant success. In this country, and the British Isles, within the last few years, not only have individual practitioners applied its remedies with equal success, but some large veterinary institutions, and most of our principal traveling equestrian troops and menageries, employ it exclusively in all diseases of their horses, experience having shown them its great value and curative power, and its immense superiority over every other method. But the inherent intricacies of the system rendered its general introduction for the cure of animals impracticable; and though, in the hands of some practitioners and some veterinary surgeons, it worked wonders enough to show its astonishing capacities, yet to the masses it has remained a sealed book

The principle of Specific Homœopathy, which has proved so efficient in popular use, we have now applied to the diseases of domestic animals, and, from numerous trials, have proved it an entire success. With this Case and Manuel every owner of stock may know every ailment among them, and can treat it successfully.

Not among the least benefits conferred by this new method is the ease and simplicity with which the proper medicine is administered. No tying, bottling, struggling, or choking are necessary. A neat little glass instrument (the Medicator) is put into the medicine, and takes up the requisite dose—a few drops—and at the proper moment, is placed in the mouth of the animal and discharged; in an instant the dose is given, and an amount of labor is thus saved to the owner, and of suffering to the animal, which is by no means trivial. Hundreds of animals annually die, or are rendered valueless from disease and drugging, that may be saved and promptly restored by the use of the Case of Veterinary Specifics. Several of our most experienced horsemen have given it their unqualified commendation, and use it daily in their establishments.

In the execution of this design I have consulted every authority and drawn upon every resource within my reach, and the experience of each has been made to contribute to the perfection of the whole, and all has been combined and compared with my now nearly twenty years of observation, study, and experience in the practice of Homœopathy. We flatter ourselves that for simplicity, completeness, and reliability it will commend itself to the judgment of a discerning public.

F. HUMPHREYS, M.D.

New York, May 18, 1860.

PREFACE.

SECOND REVISED AND ENLARGED EDITION.

It is now twelve years since the first edition of my HOMŒOPATHIC VETERINARY MANUAL was issued. At that time, the doctrine of SPECIFIC HOMŒOPATHY was less understood than now. Although the Veterinary Specifics had then been repeatedly tried in practice, yet there was a considerable degree of hesitation and embarrassment in their use, from the want of more ample experience and intimate knowledge of their curative virtues. The embarrassment and hesitancy has happily passed away. Though no special effort has been made to push them by extended advertisements, yet the VETERINARY HOMŒOPATHY SPECIFICS prepared by me have been constantly extending in use and gaining in confidence, until they are now recognized as the most simple, efficient and reliable medicines in use for the cure of the Diseases of Domestic Animals. Experience has amply demonstrated their value, and the long list of commendations appended to this volume sufficiently attest the value in which they are held by those who have long used them. These commendations come from every class of community. From professional horse-men and breeders, from Livery Stables and Horse Railroad men, from Owners and Managers of Menageries and Equestrian Troops, from gentlemen farmers, Sporting men, Horse-trainers, and Farmers, and

Newspaper Agriculturalists, and all unite in commendation of their excellence and recommendation of their use.

But few alterations have been found necessary. The doses have been rendered more uniform, and ten drops has been fixed as the standard for horses, experience having shown that while less might be sufficient, more would not be injurious, and that while the exact number cannot always be arrived at, this standard of Ten drops is the dose which should be approximated as nearly as the circumstances permit, will be found the most convenient and effective.

Several new articles have been added. Notably that upon the CANADIAN HORSE DISEASE or Epizootic of which quite full description and treatment is given. A very large experience has shown how amply those Specifics are adapted to the cure of this disease. Among the many thousands treated by them in this city and elsewhere, none so far as can be ascertained, has terminated unfavorably. And such has been the demand for them that our Books have run out and the entire energies of the establishment have been taxed to keep up with the demand.

With the additions and corrections now made, I cannot but think this Manual will more than ever commend itself to all who have the welfare of our Domestic Animals at heart, and who desire, when such have the misfortune to become sick or diseased, to have remedies on hand which are simple, convenient and efficient for their cure.

F. HUMPHREYS, M.D.

NEW YORK, NOV. 4, 1872.

PREFACE.

THIRD REVISED AND ENLARGED EDITION.

It is now nearly five years since the SECOND REVISED EDITION of this MANUAL of VETERINARY HOMEOPATHIC SPECIFICS was issued. Since that period, this system of VETERINARY HOMŒPATHIC SPECIFICS has come more and more into general use, aud a demand for a yet more complete and comprehensive work has been created. The general treatment of the diseases noted in the previous editions has been preserved, only that the doses of medicine have been somewhat increased, to conform more to popular usage and the practice of many veterinary surgeons. Still, doses are yet an open question, and the quantity given at a time is far less important than the kind of medicine. Several new sections have been added, notably those upon SPINAL MENINGITIS in horses, and on the so-called HOG CHOLERA, and a chapter on DISEASES OF POULTRY.

With these additions and annotations, we commend this manual to the attention of all engaged in the Breeding or Handling of Domestic Animals, as embodying the most plain, concise, simple, and yet effective method of treatment ever offered to the public.

F. HUMPHREYS, M. D.

New York, Sept., 1877.

INTRODUCTION.

PROPER and enlightened attention to the wants of Domestic Animals, is not only a sentiment of humanity, but a dictate of economy. To know at least in good part what is the particular ailment of an animal, and to know also how to relieve it, would seem to be a necessary obligation of ownership. The least we can return to the many faithful animals given us, is to provide for their reasonable wants, not only in health, but also sickness and disease. Not that every man who owns a horse, should be necessarily a veterinary surgeon; and yet the way is so simple that any intelligent person may readily cure a very large proportion, nay, almost every disease to which his animals are exposed, and yet bestow upon the subject only a moiety of attention.

Among the many blessings that Homœopathy has conferred upon the world, not among the least is the immense improvement which it has effected in the treatment of the diseases of Domestic Animals. With but little variation, to meet their peculiar habits and susceptibilities, the same remedies which have been so efficient in mitigating and curing the disease of men, women and children, have been found equally successful in arresting the diseases to which all classes of Domestic Animals are liable. The contrast is even greater. Probably from the fact that the treatment of sick animals has been but little understood, and intrusted to the hands mainly of ignorant persons, who have pursued the most crude, cruel and destructive measures, often far more dangerous and life destroying than the disease itself, a large proportion of the sick have died or been tortured to death. But when the same diseases are subjected to the mild and benign influence of intelligent Homœopathic treatment, it is found that almost every disease among them is within control, even the most fatal yielding to its magic influences.

Although at first sight it may seem strange, that animals should be successfully treated by the mild and apparently insignificant doses of Homœopathy, yet a moment's reflection will suffice to give many reasons why this should be so. Even were it not susceptible of explanation, experience has abundantly demonstrated the fact, that animals are, if possible, even more susceptible to Homœopathic treatment than men, and its success in their case is even more striking and brilliant.

This may be, perhaps, attributed to their more regular habits, confinement to the same food and drink, absence of excitement, and freedom from the many articles of food and drink in use among the human species, which are more or less medicinal.

Owing to these circumstances, animals are very

impressible, and the doses for them need not be so much larger than for the human species. It seems to be a law of nature, that the more delicate the organism, the more subject to disease. Wild animals are almost entirely exempt, while the highly artificial lives of some Domestic Animals render them subject to numerous ailments and to some very formidable diseases. Yet, as a whole, animals are far less subject to disease than men, and far more amendable to cure.

The treatment of Domestic Animals with SPECIFIC HOMŒOPATHIC REMEDIES, has numerous advantages.

THE MEDICINES ARE GIVEN AT ONCE and without trouble or annoyance, even without taking a horse from his team, or a cow from her stall. THEY PRODUCE NO POISONOUS OR PROSTRATING EFFECT so that the animal rallies at once, and without loss or deterioration of value. ANIMALS RECOVER MUCH SOONER and hence are able to resume work much earlier after sickness, than under any other system. But more than all, it is far more successful. Slighter diseases yield at once, and often from a single dose, while the most formidable cases of Pleuro-Pneumonia, or Founder, in horses, and Lung Murrain and Milk Fever, in cows, cases that are almost absolutely incurable under old treatment, even when well conducted, p omptly respond to the curative influence of Specific Homœopathic Remedies, while it is well known that even when animals recover under the old system of treatment, such have been the ravages of disease and medicine, that their value and usefulness are generally destroyed.

LIST OF

VETERINARY HOMEOPATHIC SPECIFICS

—AND—

SYMPTOMATIC INDICATIONS FOR THEIR USE.

A A. Cures { FEVER, INFLAMMATIONS, AND CONGESTION.

THIS Specific is especially curative for all FEVERS, febrile conditions, and *Inflammations*, and for all conditions attended with QUICK, FULL, or STRONG PULSE, HEAT, *Great Excitement of the System;* or for the *Coldness, Shaking*, or *Panting*, which precedes fever.—

In particular for :—*Coldness, Prickly Coat, Shaking* or *Panting Chill.*—

Heat of the Head and red, injected eyes.—

INFLAMMATION of the EYES, from congestion, or from something having gotten into the eye, or an injury.—

INFLAMMATION of the THROAT—QUINSY—with difficult or painful deglutition, and general fever, in alternation with C C.—

INFLAMMATION of the WINDPIPE, (Larynx), with heat, loud, stridulous whistling breathing, even with danger of suffocation.—

INFLAMMATION of the LUNGS or PLEURA, with heat of body, cold legs, painful, labored, difficult, or oppressed breathing.—

Palpitation, or loud, hurried, or unequal beating of the heart.—

INFLAMMATORY COLIC, with extreme pain; or when F F. fails to give relief, or when colic threatens to terminate in inflammation of the bowels.—

Inflammation of the *Liver* in Cattle.—

Inflammation of the *Kidney* or *Bladder*, in alternation with H H.—

HOT or RHEUMATIC *Swelling* of the *Feet* and *Legs*.—

INFLAMMATION of the FEET, with heat, extreme tenderness, difficult moving, or even standing on them.—

MILK FEVER in Cows after Calving.—

FITS, *Convulsions*, or *Staggers*,—the animal suddenly stands, falls back, or to one side, or rushes off madly, or falls down.—

The results of fear, fright, anger, or excitement.

Inflammation of the *Brain*, with heat, excitement, *frenzy*.—

Congestion of the *Head*, with dull, stupid, sleepy, hanging of the head, or its opposite stage of excitement.—

PINK EYE, with fever, heat of the head, red, or watery, or injected eyes, swelled legs, swelling under the jaw, and dull, stupid appearance; See also C C. SPINAL MENINGITIS.

SPINAL MENINGITIS in horses, with dull red or injected eyes, heavy hanging head, slow swaying, or feeble gait, painful stiff awkward turning or backing; pain on pressure along the spine or back; difficult standing, tottering or swaying about; is easily pushed over while standing, or inability to rise when down; suppressed or very scanty staling or dung.

HOG CHOLERA, so called, with dullness, weakness, don't eat, unsteady gait, buries its head or body in the straw, shiverings and feverish heat, quick pulse or breathing; bowels bound, or dung hard and dark colored; efforts to vomit; red spots or patches on the inside of the legs, belly or breast, which swell, become blood red or crimson or purple; labored breathing, heaving of flanks and cough; inability to rise in the advanced stages. See also I I.

B B. CURES

STRAINS, INJURIES, LAMENESS.

This Specific is especially curative for all diseases, affections, or morbid conditions of the MUSCULAR SYSTEM, the SINEWS, TENDONS, and JOINTS.—

More especially for:—

RHEUMATIC STIFFNESS or Lameness of the Entire System, or the forelegs, shoulder, back, or loins, or a single leg, the result of a strain, over-work, or a chill.—

Affection of the *Hock*, Knee, or Pastern, with heat, stiffness, or Lameness, resulting in spavin, splint, ring-bone, or similar defect.—

Rheumatic Lameness of the Shoulder, (shoulder sprain).—

INCIPIENT SPAVIN—bone-spavin, blood-spavin, so called, with heat and tenderness of the part, and slight or severe lameness.—

Tenderness or weakness of the Tendons, resulting in stifle or dislocation of the patella.—

Want of Synovia or joint oil, and cracking on moving the joint.—

Results of Fatigue, or of over-work.—

Lameness of any kind, or when the origin is uncertain.—

Old Chronic Founder, or lameness and stiffness on first starting.—

C C. CURES }

INFLUENZA, QUINSY, NASAL GLEET.

This Remedy is especially curative for all diseases of the mucous membrane and glandular system. Hence is especially curative for:—

INFLUENZA, with rough coat, red or watery eyes, *Sore Throat, Profuse Disharge* from the *Head*, first of thin acrid, then of copious, thick, yellow, or greenish mucus, attended with fever, great weakness or debility, swelling of the glands of the neck, or even of the head, face, throat, sheath, and limbs, or even general dropsy.—

QUINZY, or Sore Throat, with fever, heat, *Soreness* and *Swelling* of *the Throat*, difficult, *painful*, or even impossible swallowing, so that the fluid returns through the nostrils.—

Soreness of the Throat, so that the animal will not swallow, but quids his food, and splashes the water about with his nose.—

NASAL GLEET, or Strangles, with swelling and even suppuration of the glands about the neck, discharge of thick, copious matter from the nose, and general emaciation.—

D D. CURES

BOTS, GRUBS, OR WORMS.

This Specific is especially curative for all conditions or diseases arising from the various kinds of *Worms*, *Bots*, or *Grubs*, or other species of ENTOSIA in the animal system, as well as for the *morbid cause* which produces them in excess.—

In particular for:

Bots or *Grubs*, indicated by *Emaciation*, the horse losing flesh, or keeping very poor without apparent cause, enlarged or pendulent abdomen; turns of griping or colic; eating or drinking greedily.—

Appearance of Bots or Grubs hanging about the fundament, or discovered in the manure.—

Morbid Appetite; eating lime, chalk, or gnawing the wall.—

Frequent returns of Colic without apparent cause.—

General Unthriftiness, staring coat, want of spirit, and ill condition.—Easily fatigued.

E E. CURES } COUGHS, BRONCHITIS,

INFLAMED LUNGS.

This Specific is especially curative for all morbid conditions of the air-passages and Lungs, especially for:

Bronchitis or common cough, coming on after exposure, attended or not with severe pain, or even with some heat or fever.—

COUGH, without any other apparent symptom. (See also A A.)

COUGH, attended with whistling, roaring, or other difficulty of breathing.—

INFLAMMATION of the LARYNX, with loud, difficult, stirdulous breathing, (after the more violent symptoms have been removed by A A.

INFLAMMATION of the LUNGS or PLEURA, (PLEURO-PNEUMONIA), with painful, labored, difficult breathing, occasional grunting or groaning cough, heat of the body, cold ears and legs; (after or in alternation with A A.)

Difficult, painful breathing.—

Breathing intercepted or accompanied by a grunt.—

Loud whistling when hurried or driven fast.

Results of Bronchitis, Pneumonia or other badly cured affection of the lungs, or air-passages.—

ADVANCED STAGE of PLEURO-PNEUMONIA in Cattle, after the use of A A, or in alternation with that remedy.—

F F. CURES } COLIC, BELLY-ACHE, WIND-BLOWN, DIARRHEA.

This Specific is more especially adapted to the cures of the various forms of COLIC or ENTERALGIA and the derangements arising from *over-feeding, improper food,* or *deranged digestion.* Hence it is always curative for—

COLIC, SPASMODIC, or FLATULENT COLIC, with turns of terrible griping and distress, the animal pawing, rolling, lying down and getting up, straining to pass wind—and especially when occasioned by flatulent or improper food, deranged digestion or a chill; (compare also A A, for inflammatory colic).—

Hoven or *Wind-Blown,* in consequence of being gorged with clover or too succulent food in early summer. The ANIMAL IS PUFFED up like a DRUM, is terribly uneasy, or stands stupidly, passes nothing and rumination has ceased.—

Hoven or over-distention, in consequence of being gorged with grain or other improper food. See also J J.—

DIARRHEA, or too loose passages in calves, sheep, cattle, or even horses frequent passages of loose bad-colored, unnatural dung,—often attended with weakness and emaciation.—

DYSENTERY, with frequent slimy, bloody, or discolored discharges of dung, attended with constantly increasing weakness and loss of flesh.—

G G. CURES } MISCARRIAGE, IMPERFECT CLEANSING OR HEMORRHAGE.

This remedy is more especially appropriate to the diseases or morbid conditions connected with the reproductive system. Hence especially useful as a *preventive* of MISCARRIAGE or the CASTING of CALF, when it has occurred in a herd of cattle and to prevent the infection from spreading, or when *premonitory symptoms* have been observed in cows or mares.—

Retention of the placenta or imperfect cleansing in cows, mares, or other animals.—

HEMORRHAGE or FLOODING, occurring before, during, or after the delivery of the animal.

Stimulates the proper contraction of the Womb after delivery and even during labor, in delaying or tedious confinements.—

"Foolishness" or hysteria of young mares, at certain periods.—

H H. CURES } URINARY & KIDNEY DISEASES, AND DROPSY.

Especially curative for all affections of the urinary apparatus, the kidneys, bladder, and appendages.—

Particularly for:—

INFLAMMATION of the KIDNEYS with *frequent, scanty, high-colored, or even bloody urination,* or straining with passage of a few drops, or in effectual attempts at staling, heat of the loins and shrinking when pressed upon, pain in turning, back is arched and legs wide apart, or he straddles in walking, with heat and quick pulse, and anxious appearance.—

INFLAMMATION of the BLADDER, with frequent painful attempts at staling, and discharge of but a few drops of hot saturated urine, which may be clear, or mixed with *mucus,* or more commonly *bloody.*—

Constant attempts to void or pass the urine.

Too constant urination.—

Dropsy of the Belly.—

General Dropsy, Anasarca, the entire body, sheath, and limbs are swelled.—

Frequent attempts at staling, with effort or straining, and passage of but very little water.—

RENAL COLIC, or colic from irritation of the

kidneys, the horse throws himself down, rises, and threshes himself about in terrible distress, making frequent or almost constant attempts at staling, with passage of very little or trifling discharge of water.—

RETENTION of URINE, the animal can pass but little, or the urine may be almost entirely suppressed.—

BLOODY or *blood stained* urine, accompanied or not with tenderness of the loins, or lameness as if from an injury.—

DROPSY of the LEGS, SHEATH, or *along under the belly*, with scanty secretion of urine.

GENERAL DROPSY or *swelling of the face, lips, belly, sheath, legs*, and all depending portions of the body, with stiff, clumsy movements and scanty secretion of urine.

I I. CURES } ERUPTIONS, ULCERS, MANGE, GREASE, FARCY, ABSCESSES, FISTULAS, UNHEALTHY SKIN, ETC.

THIS Specific is especially applicable to all diseases of the SKIN or UNDERLYING TISSUES, to all ABSCESSES and ULCERATIONS, and the *morbid condition precedent* to their appearance.—

Hence for.—

MANGE in horses, or dogs, with violent itching, and eruption of small, bran-like scales, or of reddish pimples.—

ERYSIPELAS, with red, hot, inflamed skin, heat, swelling, and tenderness of the part.

FARCY, with buds appearing along the course of the inflamed lymphatics, with or without discharge, or ulceration, hardened lymphatics or cords, and swelling or tumefaction, pain and tenderness along the inside of the thighs, swelled legs, ulcerations, cough, great debility and emaciation. (Compare also C C.)—

GREASE or SCRATCHES, with swelling and heat, cracks, or deep clefts, discharge of thick, gummy matter, or even formation of unhealthy vegetations or grapes.—

ABSCESS or hot swellings, with a collection of matter, wherever situated.—

ULCERATIONS, either flat, superficial, or deep-seated with sinuses, pipes, or FISTULAS, burrowing deep, with narrow openings.—

FISTULAS, with narrow openings, and deep-seated or torturous ulcerations.—

WARTS, or horny appendages, or unhealty-thickening of the skin.—

UNHEALTHY SKIN, every injury tends to suppuration.—

FALLING OFF of the *hair*.—

ROUGH STARING or *unhealthy coat*.—

PLEURO-PNEUMONIA in horses or cattle, in the more advanced stages, with great prostration or sinking of strength, or in alternation with E E.—

HOG CHOLERA in the more advanced stages or malignant form, with red pimples or dark patches of the skin, ulcers or blisters, bloody discharges, great weakness and rapid failing of strength, after or in alternation with A A.

J J. CURES } INDIGESTION, SURFEIT, OVER-FEED, BAD CONDITION, PARALYSIS, STOMACH STAGGERS.

This medicine is especially applicable to all conditions arising from, or in connection with DERANGEMENTS of the DIGESTIVE SYSTEM, and morbid conditions of the cerebro-spinal system connected therewith. Hence it is especially curative for:

INDIGESTION, the mouth is slimy, the tongue foul, dung dry, or mixed with undigested oats, the horse is weak, thin, sweats easily, and does not fatten, with bad coat and hide bound skin.

Loss of APPETITE, deficient appetite, "off his feed."—

IRREGULAR APPETITE.—

CRIB BITING.—

RESULTS of OVER-FEED, the horse is dull, stupid, moves clumsily, has slimy mouth, foul tongue, scanty staling, and dry scanty dung.—

STOMACH STAGGERS, with dull, stupid, sleepy condition, scarcely moves or eats, hanging head, slow labored breathing, half closed yellowish eyes, slight convulsions, or sometimes uneasy turns as if distressed.—

BAD CONDITION, staring coat, irregular appetite, bound bowels, want of spirit, and constantly increasing emaciation.—

Staring Coat, in connection with indigestion.—

PARALYSIS of the hind legs, the animal is weak behind, sways about, totters or falls, and cannot rise, or gets out his fore-feet, but cannot rise from paralysis.—

SPINAL MENINGITIS after the more violent symptoms have yielded to A A, or, when there remains *greal debility* or *inability to rise,* or when the animal is slow in recovering the use of his limbs or his strength.

Incipient paralysis, tottering movements, swaying about.—

ILL-GROWING, *brittle, weak,* or defective hoofs.—

Defective Horny Deposit, liability to sand or quarter crack.—

In addition to the foregoing Specifics, which are all given internally, the following remedies and preparations are also employed externally as washes or applications, at the same time that the Specific remedy is also internally employed.

1. The Marvel of Healing.

This is a most invaluable application for Burns, Cuts, Bruises, Soreness, Lameness, Sprains, Saddle or Harness Galls, Boils, Ulcers, Old Sores, and Wounds. It is given to relieve local inflammation or arrest all soreness or hemorrhage. It is similar in its action to Arnica, but far more prompt and efficient. It may be applied in full strength.

2. Arnica Montana.

This medicine is used as a lotion for all kinds of injuries, Bruises, Concussions, or Strains. The tincture is prepared by adding a pint of alcohol to two ounces of the dried flowers. The lotion is prepared by adding a tablespoonful of the tincture to a pint of water.

3. Calendula Officinalis

Is used in case of lacerations, and in all flesh wounds as well as old ulcers, or when there is sloughing or considerable loss of substance. The lotion is made by adding a tablespoonful of the tincture to a pint of water. The Calendula (common Marigold) is a common and pretty flower, readily grown in gardens or plats. The plant taken during flowering and cut up and covered with alcohol, forms the mother tincture.

4. Sulphur Ointment.

Is readily prepared by rubbing intimately in a mortar one ounce of flour of sulphur with two ounces of lard. It is used for Mange and some other forms of eruption.

5. Arsenical Lotion.

Is sometimes used in cases of Mange, Cracked Heels, Grease, etc. It is prepared by boiling four grains of white arsenic (arsenious acid), in one pint of distilled water.

6. Bran Poultice.

Pour hot water over bran, and permit to stand until about milk-warm, and then apply it.

7. Turnip or Carrot Poultice.

Boil these vegetables until quite soft, then mash and apply them quite warm.

Form of Homeopathic Medicines.

Three forms are principally in use, namely, tinctures, dilutions, powders, and medicated pellets. Each have their advantages and objections, but after an extensive experience and ample survey of the entire ground we prefer for animals the low dilutions. The dose is rather more positive; and they meet on the whole every reasonable requirement.

Doses. How Much?

It is an error to suppose that animals require very large doses of SPECIFIC HOMŒOPATHIC MEDICINES, for experience has shown sick animals to be very impressible, and easily influenced by appropriate medicine, and in general, not to require as frequent repetitions as the human subject. Those who are accustomed to give large and powerful doses of poisonous medicines in order to produce some revulsive action, such as a cathartic or sudorific, or even as an alternative, can not from hence infer the proper quantity required when only a curative result is desired.

Only experience hence can answer the question, How much? And experience has amply shown that for horses ten to fifteen drops is the range of doses best adapted in ordinary cases, and that while cattle and hogs require rather more, sheep and dogs require less than the doses mentioned. We have indicated in each disease the dose supposed to be best for that particular case, yet to give two or five drops more in any given case would probably not be hurtful, while to give a few drops less would not endanger the curative action for want of the requisite quantity. The truth is that precision in quantity is not indispensable to a cure. The doses indicated we think are best, but a deviation from them is by no means fatal. One physcian gives much more and another many times less, and both are successful. Medicine gives a curative impulse often as well or better with five or ten drops as with more. Besides, in giving medicines to animals, from their restlessness, dodging the head, and other similar disturbing circumstances we can not, and happily need not, be very positive Give the doses as near the directions, as you may be able, and the result will be satisfactory. Young animals require but half as much as grown ones.

Repetitions. How Often?

The effects of Specific Homoepathic Remedies are very prompt and positive. Often immediate, in cases of colic other forms of neuraligia, as the medicine acts at once through the medium of the nervous system. In other acute cases such as inflammations, the effect is equally as prompt, but not so openly manifested. The medicine placed in contact with the nervous papilla of the tongue is at once by means of this connection conveyed over the entire system, while the stomach being a screting rather than an absorbing surface rather repells than absorbs a medicinal influence so that medicines usually act better from being placed on the tongue, than when they are introduced into the stomach.

After a dose of medicine has been given and good results are being manifested—the animal easier, more quite and apparently relieved, it is wise not to interfere with even a new dose until that good action is exhausted. *Hence the time to repeat, is when that good effect has terminated.* All rules of repetition are based upon this axiom. Thus, in colic and inflamma tion of the bowels, we repeat every fifteen, thirty, or sixty minutes. In inflammation of the lungs, or chest, head, or other noble organ, or in pneumonia or similar acute diseases, we repeat once in two, three, or four hours. In the yet less severe forms of disease such as Fevers, Founder, Strangles, Distemper, Lameness, or similar diseases, a dose once in four hours, or four times per day, is quite sufficient. While in Coughs, Heaves, Ulcers, Eruptions, and similar affections, if recent a dose morning and night is ample. In old chronic affections, a dose every day, or every second day, is better than more frequent repetitions, and in not a few cases a single dose of medicine never repeated, has cured an old, long standing and obstinate disease.

Alternation of Remedies.

In general but one medicine is required for a disease, and it may be repeated from time to time, until the case is cured. But cases are often so constituted that two Specifics are indicated at the same time, one to meet one phase of the disease, and a different specific to meet another. In all such cases the two medicines may be given alternately with great propriety and advantage. Thus, give a dose of one Specific. and then, after the proper interval has elapsed, give the other one, and thus continue the two alternately, at such intervals as the directions or exigencies of the case demand. Nor should we be deterred from the use of a specific in a particular case, because the name given it indicates a different use, for a medicine may be curative or specific for a particular disease, and equally so for a very different or even seemingly opposite one. Colic and Scarlet Fever are very different diseases, yet Belladonna frequently cures both.

How to Choose the Remedy.

In the use of the Homœopathic Specifics nothing can be more simple than the choice of the Remedy, while in attempting to use the ordinary Homœopathic preparations, the choice of the remedy is very difficult and intricate. From an examination of the animal you will have some idea of the nature of its disease, and will at once turn to the Index and page in the Manual describing that and similar diseases, and continue the search until the true description is found, and the proper treatment will be pointed out. It is not necessary that all the symptoms given in the description should be present in each case, it will be sufficient if a general outline of them are present, as the Specific will in all cases be found to have a much wider range of action than the single disease or symptoms required.

In case a wrong medicine is selected or given, no injury will be done, only a possible loss of time may result.

And when a sufficient length of time has passed to clearly show that no good has resulted, the case should be looked over again, and a more appropriate Specific selected.

How to give the Remedy.

Not among the least recommendations for the use of these Homœopathic Specifics, is the ease and facility with which they may be administered. No tying, struggling, or choking are necessary. The animal should be approached quietly, usually on the OFF SIDE if the Medicator is to be used, and medicine placed, if possible, upon the tongue, well back—thence it is absorbed, and acts through the medium of the nervous system. The simplest method of doing this is best. For this purpose I prefer the use of the Medicator—a small glass instrument invented by me. It is about five inches in length, made of firm, heavy glass tubing, (see plate page,) the lower third bent so as to enter the mouth with facility, and terminating in a fine orifice. The upper end funnel-shaped the size of the end of the finger, and covered with an air-tight rubber-cap, so as to form an air receiver. The Medicator, taken in the right hand, with the fore-finger upon the top or rubber valve, is introduced into the proper vial, and pressing slightly upon the valve the air is exhausted, and on removing the finger the fluid is forced up into the tube sufficient for a dose. A little experience will enable one to take up five, ten or more drops as may be required. The Medicator thus charged with the dose, can, at the convient moment, be inserted just within the lips of the animal's mouth, the farther back upon the tongue the better, when a slight pressure upon the top of the tube injects the contents, and the medicine is given.

THE MEDICATOR should be held upright; never turned down or held horizontally, as the air is thus introduced and the medicine may drop out. Held upright until it is quietly inserted between the lips of the animal, no such difficulty obtains. Nor is it necessary to push the tube far enough into the mouth to expose it to the danger of being broken or crushed between the teeth. The moment the fluid from the tube comes upon the tongue the animal will open the mouth, and in an instant the medicine is injected upon the tongue or in the mouth, and the operation is finished.

In other cases the tongue may be gently hooked out of the mouth with the finger, and the medicine may be dropped or turned upon it. Horses are fond of sugar, and the medicine may be dropped upon a small lump, and fed from hand. After a few times they will call for their sugar, when the owner comes into the stable, at the proper time. With cattle or sheep, raise the head a little, and inject the medicine with the Medicator, or pull the tongue out on one side, and drop or eject the medicine upon it.

When quite a number of animals are to receive the same medicine, it is better to drop out the quantity for all in a proper bowl or other vessel, and add a spoonful of water for each dose to the medicine. Then stir well the entire mass, and give a spoonful, or other proportionate quantity, to each. Hogs usually, when sick, lie quietly upon the side, and the medicine may hence be injected into the mouth with the Medicator, or it may be given in a spoonful of sweet milk, poured in between the jaws, or it may be given them to drink. Care must be taken in giving fluid to hogs, not to forcibly raise the head, as they are thus easily strangled—even to death. Dogs may have the medicine in a little sweet milk, or it may be even turned in through the nose. Yet the Medicator is an improvement upon all these plans, as it takes up and discharges the proper dose at once.

N. B.—Take off the rubber cap, and cleanse the Medicator when using it for different medicines or specifics.

Housing and Care of Sick Animals.

When an animal shows signs of illness, it should be immediately cared for. The horse, unless in cases of Colic, or other slight ailment, when the medicine may be given at once, and his work continued, should be placed in a roomy, convenient and warm stall, well littered, with plenty of dry bedding, and well blanketed, unless in very warm weather. Cattle, sheep, and hogs, as soon as it is noticed that they are sick, should be separated from the herd or flock, and placed in a comfortable and well-littered and especially dry apartments. This is necessary not only to prevent disease spreading to other stock on the farm, but for the convenience of nursing them, giving them medicines, but also to place them in the very best position for a cure. Often a little timely care and nursing will save and restore an animal, which, if permitted to run with the stock, and take its chance, would unquestionably be lost. A sick animal as truly needs attention as a sick child. Not always will mere nursing restore a sick animal, but it always places it in the best possible condition to effect a cure, and without it the best medical treatment will often be fruitless.

Diet of Sick Animals.

In general, when animals are seriously ill, they are without appetite, and will take little or no food—nature thus indicating the propriety of abstinence. But in all cases the food given or allowed should be quite limited in quantity—one-half, one-third or fourth of the usual quantity, and only that which is nourishing easily digested, and generally relaxing. With these general restrictions, the usual kinds of food may be permitted, except in case of dogs, where *only stale bread and milk* should be allowed in urgent cases, and but little or no meat, and no salted or spiced food in any case. After the more urgent symptoms of disease have passed over, and the animal is recovering, we should be careful and not give full feed, as a relapse may thus easily be provoked, and prove very stubborn and dangerous.

At least half an hour or hour should intervene after taking a dose of medicine, before the animal should be fed, as the system is more susceptible then than at any other time.

All nostrums, domestic medicines, or herb-teas, however harmless or beneficial otherwise, are strictly prohibited, as the Specific Medicine must be permitted to act upon the system entirely undisturbed by any such prejudicial influences.

Injections of water, soap and water, or salt and water are always allowable, and may often be used with great benefit. They are usually administered without difficulty, in no case injurious, and should one fail to produce an evacuation, another or more may be repeated, until the result is accomplished.

How to Feel the Pulse.

This is best done by placing the finger on the artery, where it passes over the lower jaw, about four inches below its angle. Place the forefinger on the side of the lower jaw at its angle, and trace the jaw along gently towards the mouth. Some four inches below the angle a notch will be fouud, in which the artery passes over the jaw, and the throbbing of the pulse will be readily felt. Some attention may be required as the pulse beats in health slowly, and often apparently indistinctly.

The pulse makes in the healthy horse from thirty-six to forty-two beats per minute ; in spirited lighter horses the latter, and in heavy older horses the former. When the pulse reaches fifty to fifty five, there is some degree of fever. Seventy-five will indicate a dangerous condition, and few horses will long survive a pulse of one hundred. Care should be taken not to excite a horse before or while examining the pulse, as it may thus readily be increased ten or fifteen beats to the minute, and mislead as to the true condition.

PART I.
DISEASES OF HORSES.

CHAPTER I.

DISEASES OF THE SKIN AND SUBJACENT TISSUE.

Abscess—Ulcers.

An abscess is a collection of matter. Any tumor softening, or in other words coming to a head, forms an abscess. They are usually the result of injuries, such as a blow or contusion, or may be occasioned by a thorn, nail or splinter entering the flesh. In the more severe cases these act in connection with a constitutional pre-disposition or peculiar state of the blood.

Symptoms.—A hot and painful swelling; in the earlier stage, hard, and by degrees softening or fluctuating in the centre, and gradually approaching the surface, attended with more or less heat and fever, according to its situation and nature

Abscesses which penetrate deeply along the sheaths of muscles and tendons, or even to the bones are termed fistulas. Shallow abscesses are known as ulcers, and these may be mild, readily healing, and secreting a healthy, thick, cream-like pus; or ill-conditioned, unhealthy, secreting a thin sanious discolored matter, and healing with great difficulty.

Such are the general characteristics of all abscesses, wherever located, and their situation and extent mark their relative importance and danger.

TREATMENT.—During the inflammatory stage or before softening, while there is merely a hard, more or less hot and painful tumor, we should endeavor to disperse it without its softening. To this end, give three times per day, ten drops of the Specific, A A, for INFLAMMATION, and also bathe the tumor as often with THE MARVEL which will frequently disperse it.

But if the swelling increases and fluctuates, or a yellowish spot is observed in its centre, denoting the presence of matter, it should be lanced at once, in the most depending portion, and the matter drawn off, and fifteeen drops of the Specific, I I, for ULCERS be given morning and night to facilitate the healing. If the part is so situated that a compress wet with THE MARVEL or Calendula Lotion can be applied or bound on it, it will facilitate the healing.

The treatment of ulcers is the same.

Abscess of the Poll, Poll Evil.

Is often from neglect a very formidable disease. It is generally the result of severe injury upon the top of the head, such as the chafing of the bridle or halter, pressure, or a blow against the manger or stall, or frequent hanging back against the headstall.

SYMPTOMS.—At first a tumor forms at the polls or junction of the head and neck. It soon becomes hot, tense and painful; the horse carries his head low;

looks to one side; eats but little from the pain of chewing, especially if the food is hard. If the tumor is not dispersed, it comes to a head, either discharges externally, or the matter failing to come to the surface, sinks downward, burrowing along beneath the surface among tendons, ligaments, and bones, forming deep and obsinate fistulous ulcers

TREATMENT.—Before the tumor has softened, give the Specific A A, for INFLAMMATION, fifteen drops three times per day, keep the horse on low diet, and bathe the swelling frequently with the Marvel or the Arnica Lotion. This course will usually disperse the swelling or should it fail to do so, will limit it to the smallest possible extent

If the tumor has come to a head, is soft or fluctuating, lance it at once, evacute the contents, and give fifteen drops of the Specific I I, for ULCERS, morning and night, bathing the ulcer with the MARVEL or the CALENDULA LOTION from time to time, to facilitate its healing. If already discharging, proceed as after having opened it.

Allopecia, or Falling off of the Hair.

Sometimes in animals the hair falls off either in patches or generally. If it is attended with itching and irritation, consult what is said under the head of MANGE, but in most cases the disease may be arrested, and the hair restored by giving a dose of fifteen drops of the Specific I I, for ERUPTION, each morning and night for a few days. The loss of hair may be soon arrested, but new growth will be slow.

Anasarca—Dropsy.

This disorder, which is often a mere extension of dropsy of some other part of the system, but may also occur alone, consists of collection of serum in the cellular tissue immediately beneath the skin. It may be known by the *doughy* feel of the part, the pit made by pressure retaining for a time the impression made, and it is usually accompanied by scanty urination, dry skin, and other symptoms of dropsy.

It will generally be cured by giving the SPECIFIC H H, in doses of fifteen drops three times per day for trifling cases, or ten drops every three hours for the more severe ones. After a free discharge of urine is established, giving the medicine three times per day will be sufficient.

Antichor.

Is the name given to a globular inflammatory swelling, sometimes the size of the fist, which occasionally forms on the chest opposite the heart. It is a consequence of cold and straining, and will yield to a few doses of fifteen drops each of the SPECIFIC A A, for FEVER, repeated three times per day.

Exanthemes.

There are various forms of Exanthematous diseases to which men and animals are subject, and which have been most elaborately arranged and classified by writers who have devoted themselves to this particular subject. They are, however, of little value to us in a practical point of view, as these distinctions are often too intricate to be followed by the amature, and lead to no practical difference in the treatment. They may be ACUTE or CHRONIC, DRY or SCURVY and attended with ITCHING and BURNING; or MOIST and SECRETING matter.

These are all treated by internal remedies, and with scarcely any external applications, and experience has abundantly shown that this mode of treatment is far less troublesome, as well as more safe, than that of external washes and applications. Every eruptive disease is only the manifestation of an internal morbid condition, and requires only the cure of that morbid condition in order to its entire disappearance externally.

Old School Homœopathy offers a great variety of medicines for different forms of exanthemata, but my Specific, I I, will be found applicable to all of them, with scarce an exception, and the use of it in any eruptive disease is a mere question of dose and repetition.

For PIMPLES *which form on the surface*, scale off and fall in a powder or scurf, give fifteen drops of the ERUPTION SPECIFIC, I I, every night and morning

For dry eruptions, with disequamation or branny scaling off of the skin, give the same dose and repetition.

For Sudden Itching after a cold, the same.

Moist eruptions, where there are blisters, (vesicles) or pustules which rise above the skin, break and secrete a fluid which is poured upon the surface, forming crusts and scabs, and is attended with very troublesome itching, require a dose of fifteen drops of the same Specific, I I, three times a day. In any form of eruption attended with heat, burning and great uneasiness, the dose should be given more frequently, and to relieve the anguish and fever, a few doses of the FEVER SPECIFIC, A A, may be given from time to time between the doses of I I, with most excellent effect.

Fistulas.

Abscesses which have a small opening, with a straight or sinuous canal, burrowing along beneath the surface, among the muscles, tendons, sheaths, and even bones, are called FISTULAS. They are distinguished according to their location, extent, and general characteristics, as follows:

FISTULA in the NECK, or Poll Evil; fully described in a preceding page, under that head.

VENOUS FISTULA, from inflammation along the course of a vein, from blood-letting.

FISTULA IN ANO; from docking too near the anus, and improper treatment.

FISTULA of the CORONA; generally on the inner side of the corona or frog of the foot, and if the disease lasts some time, the entire hoof becomes affected and altered, the animal becomes lame, and walks upon the toe.

SALIVARY FISTULA; which sometimes occurs in the salivary duct, where it passes round the edge of the posterior jaw.

FISTULA of the WITHERS; which is situated where the neck and back unite, and is of the most formidable character, and may even endanger the life of the animal, from the pus sinking down and extending to vital parts beneath.

DENTAL FISTULA, on the lower border of the lower jaw, sometimes on the outer surface, is frequently very painful, so that the animal refuses to eat and grows thin.

The above are the more common forms of Fistula, and the general character, causes, and treatment, are much the same, wherever located.

CAUSES.—In almost all cases, Fistulas are the result of some external injury, such as a *blow*, *strain*, *chafing*, *pressure*, etc , which, acting upon some dyscrasia or predisposition of the system, results in inflammation, suppuration, abscess and subsequent burrowing to a fistulous opening.

TREATMENT.—In case there is heat and feverish irritation, the FEVER SPECIFIC A A, should be given a few times, in doses of fifteen drops, three times per day, after which the Specific for ULCERS, FISTULAS, etc ,I I, should be given, in like doses every night and morning, except that in very old cases one dose every day is better.

In cases where the canal is long and crooked, or runs into cavities of pus, it must be laid open with the scalpel, so as to heal from the bottom. This is best done by passing a grooved probe along the canal then running a bistoury along this groove, thus laying it open to the surface. The ulcer must be kept clean, and if deep cavities exist, pressure upon the sides will much facilitate their union from the bottom by causing adhesion All such fistulous ulcers are slow in healing, and require care and attention, but with such care and management the treatment will be successful. They should be kept clean and dressed daily with the Calendula Lotion, prepared as noted on page 27, to facilitate the healing.

Grease or Scratches.

The skin of the heels of a horse has this peculiarity, that in a healthy state it secretes a greasy or oily matter which lubricates the surface, and renders it soft and pliable as well as protects it in a measure from dirt and moisture. Often, however, from want of attention, and especially in coarse animals, fever intervenes, the secretion is arrested, and the skin becomes tense and dry, red, and scurfy. The action of the joint being continued, cracks or fissures form in the skin, and a liquid is discharged profusely from the pores of the heel, at first clear like water, then thicker, turbid, greasy, corroding the skin and roots of the hair. The inflammation and pain make rapid progress; the animal cannot bear the slightest touch, limps in walking, and when at rest holds the foot off the ground. Swelling, heat, dryness, redness are the first stage; profuse moisture, cracks, and deep clefts, the second. Sometimes, in very bad and neglected cases, a yet more serious stage ensues. The ulcerations extend over the entire heel and fetlock, and in the deep clefts, which occur, and gradually extending out over the surface, *fungi* spring up, which are unhealthy vegetations and are highly sensitive, readily bleeding at the slightest touch, and interspersed with scabs. Gradually these vegetations are covered with crusts or a horny substance, protruding in the form of knots, and collected together in bunches, termed GRAPES. A fetid and peculiar exhalation arises from almost the whole of this unnatural substance. The horse suffers much, and is gradually worn down by the unnatural drain.

CAUSES.—Almost invariably the disease may be traced to want of proper care and attendance, permiting the horse to stand for days in his own litter, or his legs covered with mud; irregular work, legs much exposed to wet and mud; or working in water; add to this a tendency in some animals and families of horses to this disease. In these cases the tendency to the ulcerative form is very strong.

TREATMENT.—Regard must be had to cleanliness and diet. Remove the hair from the sores, and cleanse them well with soap and water. In bad cases the application of a bran-poultice as noticed on page 28, cleanses them beautifully. Keep the legs as dry as possible. Feed with relaxing or green food, bran-mashes, and less stimulating food, especially in the early stage, and give fifteen drops of the Specific for ERUPTIONS I, I, each morning and night If the horse is hot, feverish, or restless, give the Specific for FEVER, A A, between times a dose each foreoon and afternoon. Keep the limb as free from dirt as possible, if the horse is not worked, let him have excercise daily. For an application HUMPHREYS WITCH HAZEL OIL, is the best, simply apply it with the finger morning and night.

When *grapes have formed*, that is, unhealthy vegetations have sprouted out in deep cracks, occasional poultices of turnip or bran are useful to cleanse the part, after which apply with a brush dilute sulphuric acid to the sores Ten drops to half gill of water is strong enough, after which apply the WITCH HAZEL OIL.

CRACKED HEELS is but another form of the same disease, and requires the same treatment.

Fungus.

Is a term often applied to indurations or hardened places in the skin, occasioned by the strong and continued pressure of harness. Bathe them in THE MARVEL, night and morning, or in diluted Arnica, and give the Specific for ERUPTIONS, I I, night and morning, a dose of fifteen drops. Fungus excresences about the foot require the same treatment.

Induration of the Skin.

Hardening and tightness of the skin, when it is not the result of chafing of the harness, or external pressure, will yield to the alternate use of the Specific for ERUPTIONS I I, and that for INDIGESTION, J J, a dose of fifteen drops repeated morning and night, giving the J J, at night and the I I, mornings.

If the induration is the result of chafing or pressure, bathe the part daily with the Marvel, or Arnica, and use the medicines mentioned above internally one dose daily in alternation.

Hidebound.

This condition is not a disease of itself, but a mere symptom of some other disease, most frequently of the stomach; such as a disordered stomach; poor food, or long exposure to rough stormy weather. It not unfrequently exists in connection with Glanders, Grease, Founder or old disease of the lungs.

SYMPTOMS.—It manifests itself by the hair looking rough and unthrifty, without its natural smoothness and gloss; and the skin feels hard, firm, and fixed to the flesh.

We can most successfully treat it by ascertaining and removing the cause upon which it depends. But in the absence of any special indication, we may give with the best success a dose of fifteen drops of the Specific for INDIGESTION, J J, each morning, and the same of the Specific for ERUPTIONS, I I, each night. A few days treatment will generally produce a most marked improvement.

Mange, or Itch.

This disease, which occurs in all domestic animals, especially the horse, sheep, and dog, much resembles and is probably the same as the itch in the human subject. It may be dry and pimpled, or vesicular and moist. It first appears on the neck at the roots of the mane, thence to the back, loins, neck, buttocks, shoulders, thighs, etc., and consists of small pimples itching violently, and causing the animal to scratch and rub itself incessantly, thus soon denuding the parts. In the dry variety, the parts seem covered with a whitish dust, and the eruption constantly spreads more and more. The moist variety, consists of pimples, changing at times to pustules, which break and discharge a fluid, forming crusts or scabs, which peel off, leaving bare and sore spots. This process extends by degrees, and is attended with intolerable itching and irritation, until the entire system is more or less involved.

The animal grows thin in spite of good appetite, and unless cured, mange may continue for years, terminating fatally in some form of disease, such as dropsy, consumption, etc,

Old, badly-kept horses, and emaciated cows are especially liable to it. Sheep have it in a variety of forms. Among hogs it is quite common and most readily cured, while it is most obstinate in the case of dogs.

It is a decidedly infectious disease, and among horses is generally the result of infection, being communicated by the curry comb, brush, blanket, or by rubbing the same stall with an infected animal.

It may also arise spontaneously from spoiled or scanty food, or from damp stables, bad keeping, and poor attendance.

TREATMENT.—The horse should be so kept as not to communicate his disease to others, and be most carefully groomed and attended with a suitable allowance of good diet, and morning and night give fifteen drops of the Specifie, I, I, for MANGE. Procure also one or two pounds of good flour of Sulphur, and constantly dust this in the curry comb, brush, and cloth, used about the horse, and also in obstinate cases a table-spoonful may be stirred in a bucket of water and given daily. A wash of soap-suds, sulphur, and water may be applied every two or three days to accelerate the cure. If any ointment is deemed necessary, the sulphur ointment as described on page 28, is the best. Keep the mercurials away from the horse In obstinate cases the Arsenical lotion carefully prepared as directed on page 28, may be applied daily for three days, and then intermit for a week, and again apply the lotion if needful.

Swelled Legs.

This affection is of frequent occurrence in horses, and is more especially observed in coarse and badly groomed animals The hind legs are most subject to it, although it frequently extends to the fore legs. Sometimes from metastasis of disease from other parts, the legs swell to an enormous degree, and it is attended with some degree of heat' tenderness, and peculiar lameness. The pulse is quickened, and there is evident fever. In such cases there is some inflamation of the cellular tissue, and an effusion of fluid forming the swelling. In these cases when there is heat and tenderness, a few doses of fifteen drops each of the Specific A A, for Fever will soon relieve the lameness and swelling. If the legs are swelled without being lame or painful, the Specific, I I, for ERUPTIONS, should be given morning and night, with careful grooming and exercise will soon reduce the swelling. If the swelling is accompanied with Scanty Urination the Specific H H, fifteen drops given three times per day will promptly remove the difficulty. Sometimes swelled legs are merely the result of a change of feed, and hence often occur in spring and fall, or when horses are taken from pasture and confined in close stables. Consult also GREASE OR SCRATCHES.

Malanders and Salanders.

Scurfy eruptions sometimes appear in the bend of the knee and at the anterior bend of the hock, which after a time are attended with oozing out of mucus and formation of crust and cracks in the skin. When occurring on the fore-legs they are termed Malanders, and when on the hind legs, Salanders They produce itching, pain, and occasionally lameness. It is caused by long traveling on bad roads, want of cleanliness, and an internal virus or predisposition to the disease.

Give the Specific for ERUPTIONS, I I, in doses of fifteen drops night and morning, and if necessary bathe the part with THE MARVEL. It is usually soon relieved.

Swelling of the Teats.

Sometimes from cold or injury, the teats in mares are subject to inflammatory swelling. A few doses, ten drops each, of FEVER Specific, A A, will relieve, and if the parts seem quite tender, bathe them with the MARVEL of HEALING.

Sweating.

Sometimes, on very moderate exercise, horses sweat to excess. It is often the result of weakness, poor food or some internal condition. Give the Specific for INDIGESTION, J J, a few times in doses of fifteen drops morning and night. It will generally relieve.

Tetters.

Are sometimes met with in the horse. They consist of numerous small pimples clustered together, which after a time break and run together, forming a crust or scab devoid of hair. It is attended with itching, causing the animals to scratch. The Specific for ERUPTIONS, I I, given morning and night, in doses of fifteen drops, will be found effective.

Surfeit.

This is not an uncommon disease in horses, and arises from some obscure internal condition, in connection with the sudden changes in the kind and quality of his food; such as violent exersise or over heating; checked sweating in a draught of air; drinking cold water after work; or sudden changes in the weather. It is similar to the NETTLE RASH in people produced by similar causes and runs a similar course.

There are two forms; the *first* attended with great itching of the skin compelling the animal constantly to rub himself; the hair becomes rubbed off in several places, which are covered with a bloody scurf, or fluid of a reddish color; the skin in other places is warmer than in health; the hair is rough and unthrifty; the legs are perhaps swelled, and the horse becomes dull and weak.

In the second form, there appear upon the skin many small and hard, or large and flat lumps or swellings, which go away as quickly as they come. They may come over the whole body or only on the neck, quarters, sides, and shoulders. In other respects the animal seems well.

TREATMENT.—Give the Specific for ERUPTIONS, I, I, fifteen drops each morning, and fifteen drops of the Specific for INDIGESTION, J J, each night. A few doses will generally cure.

Tumors, Swellings.

Any unusual or morbid growth or enlargement may be termed a Tumor, and when one is found upon any part of an animal, care should be taken to ascertain, if possible, its nature and cause. They are variously named, according to their locality and the nature of their contents.

Sometimes they are globular or conical, or again flattened, or again pedunculated, (having a neck). Some are quite firm and hard, others spongy, and others contain fluid.

The principal varieties are *abdominal tumor*, which extends along the abdomen, and should not be confounded with dropsy or with pregnancy.

Tumor of the chest, which in case of the horse, is situated over the heart, is about the size of a fist, and is hot and painful. (See Antichor).

Swelling of the feet, is common among cattle and horses, and may be either hot or cold.

Swelling of the scrotum, accompanied with fever, is hot, and is liable to produce unpleasant consequences.

Swelling of the head may occur in various portions and degrees.

Swelling of the Sheath, which may become indurated by neglect.

Tumor at the point of the elbow, which is of various sizes, globular, and may attain the size of a child's head, is soft and somewhat hot. It is caused by the pressure of the shoe or by an uneven pavement while lying. After a time it becomes pendant, cold, insensible, and filled with yellowish fluid.

Tumors may form upon the edge of the eyelids, from some internal cause.

Encysted Tumors (so called because the enlargement is closed in a sack) are frequent, more or less round, movable beneath the skin. painless, and sometimes attain to a considerable size. They are the result of some internal cause not easily defined.

TREATMENT.—In all cases where a tumor or swelling is hot or painful, give the FEVER SPECIFIC, A, A, every two, four or six hours, in doses of fifteen drops according to the urgency of the case. Keep the animals on low diet and thus seek to disperse it. If caused by an external pressure or injury, bathe the part frequently with THE MARVEL, or with diluted ARNICA. If the tumor notwithstanding the treatment, has softened, grows whitish at some point, painful, and smaller, open it, then treat it as in case of an ulcer. giving the Specific for ULCERS, I I, morning and night, until healed.

In case of *cold tumors*, or hot tumors, after the heat has been reduced, simply give the SPECIFIC for Ulcers, I I, at night, or noon and night, and the CONDITION SPECIFIC J J, in the morning, in doses of fifteen drops, until the tumor is dispersed or the condition favoring the production is destroyed. Encysted and fatty tumors will generally have to be taken out by the knife, and the skin again neatly brought together and healed to prevent a scar. TUBERCLES, as they are called, are only small tumors called into existence by cold, heat, cold drinking, and other circumstances acting upon a susceptible condition of the system.

Warts.

Warts are so well known as to require no description. Certain horses and young animals are most subject to them. They vary in size and appearance, are smooth or shaggy, pedunculated or have a large base, and some are soft, moist, spongy. They sometimes arise after chafing or an injury, but depend essentially upon an internal cause.

The ERUPTION Specific, I I, given in dose of fifteen drops every two or three days, for a few weeks, should cause their entire disappearance.

Vermin.

Animals occasionally are subject to insects which fasten upon the skin and occasion great annoyance from the itching they occasion. Horses after having run out for winter, on being taken up in spring in poor condition with long rough coat, almost invariably are troubled with them. They are best and most safely destroyed by an infusion of tobacco water, after which cleanliness is only required. A dose or two of the Specific for Eruptions, I I, will also be of value as promoting the health of the skin and the growth of the hair.

CHAPTER II.

MECHANICAL INJURIES, SPRAINS, ETC.

Burns and Scalds.

BURNS occasionally occur in domestic animals. THE MARVEL may be applied directly to the surface if at hand, and is the best remedy but if not at hand, tincture of URTICA URENS and water, half and half; but if not obtainable, a soap-plaster applied to the spot relieves as promply as any other domestic remedy, and has this recommendation, that it can always be obtained. In extensive burns, give the FEVER SPECIFIC, A A, internally, fifteen drops every hour at first, then every two hours. For the ulcerations and sores resulting from burns, the Witch Hazel Oil applied night and morning, is both prompt and infallible.

Castration.

After this operation, a dose or two of the FEVER SPECIFIC, A A, is of great value to prevent fever and relieve the effects of fright, fear, &c. The parts should also be washed with THE MARVEL, or Arnica and water, to arrest inflammation and swelling, and promote healing.

Contusions.

Contusions often occur in animals from blows, kicks, falls, chafing, etc. The place exhibits either an open wound, or a swelled, black and blue appearance, and in many instances, if neglected, inflammation and suppuration may occur, and an abscess be the result. Violent shocks or contusions, when internal parts are injured, sometimes present but little appearance of injury externally, yet fever, inflammation, or other serious effects, may show themselves. Contusions about the head, and those that involve joints and bones, are most dangerous.

TREATMENT.—For all injuries, sprains, and contusions, apply THE MARVEL OF HEALING, if it can be obtained, wetting the part with it from time to time. This soon disperses the swelling and inflammation, relieves the soreness, and prevents bad consequences. Arnica is very similar, and to be used in the same manner, yet the MARVEL is preferable.

In cases where the injury has been accompanied with fright or fear, or is at all extensive, or there is reason to suspect internal organs are involved, give fifteen drops of the SPECIFIC, A A, for FEVER, and repeat the dose two or three times, at intervals of four hours, and especially so in all cases where fever is actually present. Then give the Specific for STRAINS and INJURIES, B B, repeating the remedy every two, four, or six hours, according to the urgency of the case. In the most severe cases with serious injury and high fever, the two remedies may be given alternately every hour at first, then at longer intervals.

Chafing of the collar, or girth, or saddle, only requires the MARVEL or Arnica, with which the part should be bathed from time to time, and the Specific for INJURIES, B B, may be given internally.

The result of old injuries, also, will be much benefitted by giving the Specific, B B, occasionally. Almost every possible form of injury is met by this most invaluable specific.

Capped Elbow.

This is a swelling formed at the point of the elbow, consisting of an infiltration of bloody serum, and thickened skin. It may be the result of a blow, but is most generally caused by the horse in so lying, that the calks of the shoe press upon the elbow joint. In some cases, inflammatory action sets in, and the tumor softens and is discharged, or if the pressure is continued, the swelling becomes hard and firm.

TREATMENT.—When the injury is recent, foment it with hot water three times per day, and after each fomentation apply the MARVEL or Arnica. Alter the shoe by removing the calks and smoothing the shoe, as far as possible, to prevent any further irritation. Should it have become soft, and matter formed, it should be treated as an abscess.

Capped Hock.

This form of injury most frequently results from kicking, or some similar violence, and manifests itself either as a swelling at the point of the hock, which consists of an effusion of bloody serum and thickened skin; or the swelling bulges out on each side of the hock, making the enlargement more prominent at the sides. This is found to consist of an enlargement of the bursa or small bags, which contain the lubricating fluid for the part, and over which the sinews glide.

TREATMENT.—Give the Specific, B B, for INJURIES, ten drops three times per day. Foment the part with hot water, morning and night, applying the MARVEL after each fomentation, as for capped elbow. After the heat and irritation are reduced, careful hand-rubbing will do much to disperse the enlargement of the bursa in the second form.

Curb.

At the back of the hock, three or four inches below its point, an enlargement or swelling arises, which has received the name of *curb*. It is a strain of the ring-like ligament which binds the tendons in their place, or of the sheath itself. It comes on in consequence of a violent strain of the flexor tendons, or may occur in consequence of a blow, kick, or contusion upon the part. It is most likely to occur in cow-hocked horses, where the hocks are turned inward, and the legs form a considerable angle outward, as in such cases the annular ligament must be continually on the stretch in order to confine the tendon.

When it first occurs, the swelling may not be great, but is attended with warmth, pain, and lameness, the leg being moved with caution and awkwardly.

TREATMENT.—In recent cases, bathe the part with the MARVEL or ARNICA and water often, give the horse rest, and administer the Specific, B B, for SPRAIN, fifteen drops three times per day. Continue the application of the Marvel or Arnica so long as the heat and swelling remain. Give the horse rest, for in no case is rest more absolutely required for a permament cure than in this. If prematurely put to hard labor it is very likely to return again. If the curb is permitted to run its course, the acute stage will pass off leaving a hard, cold, tumor, which may or may not materially interfere with the motion of the joint. All old cases require the Specific, B B, for SPRAIN, once or twice daily. and its continued use for some weeks, in doses of fifteen drops.

Docking.

By docking the tail of a horse, his shape and external appearance are often improved, yet the operation is not without its consequences, such as inflammation, nervous irritation, fistulous ulcers, tetanus, etc.

After the operation, bathe the part in THE MARVEL, or ARNICA, and then tie a lint saturated with it, firmly around the dock, which should be kept wet with the MARVEL until the wound is healed. This will allay all local irritation. Give first fifteen drops of the Specific, A A, for FEVER, and after a few hours, the same of the Specific, B B, for INJURIES, which may be repeated from time to time, to relieve the soreness and inflammation, and promote healing.

Fistula of the Withers.

In the article on FISTULAS, the nature and general treatment of all forms of Fistulas are given. This form of Fistula, is perhaps, more important from its location, and the nature of the structures involved. Repeated friction, or long continued compression on the withers, may injure the muscular and ligamentous parts, and give rise to a painful swelling, which, if not speedily relieved or appropriately treated, may terminate in an abscess, which, failing to come to the surface, may sink more and more among the ligaments and cartilages, extending to the very bones of the spine.

TREATMENT.—When the difficulty is still fresh, the swelling may be dispersed by applying the MARVEL, to the implicated surface, and giving fifteen drops of the Specific, A A, for FEVER three times per day. But if matter has formed, it must be opened at its lowest point, and the matter evacuated, and the Specific for ULCERS, I, I, given morning and night in doses of fifteen drops. Consult also the article on FISTULAS.

Fractures.

Fractures of the bones of the horse occasionally occur in consequence of some severe blow, contusion, fall, or other injury. They are discoverable from the *difference in shape*, the *swelling*, *lameness of the part*, and especially by the "CREPITUS," or grating sound, which occurs from moving the two fractured ends of bone together. In all doubtful cases, this crepitation is the reliable criterion. In the more palpable cases, the distortion, loss of the use of the part, and extensive swelling, remove all doubt.

Among the most common are fractures of the ribs, forming a swelling over the place, which is very sensitive to pressure. Of the pelvis, rendering one hip lower than the other. Of the leg, rendering movement and use of the limb impossible, the point below the fracture swinging about useless.

Fractures are *simple* where a single break occurs in one bone, *compound* when the surrounding parts are lacerated, and *comminuted* when bones are broken up or fractured in different directions.

The treatment of all fractures rest upon very simple principles. Bring the broken parts to their natural position, and keep them there until they unite, and the more perfectly this is done, the more perfect will be the result. Unfortunately, from the weight of the animal, and often his intractability, this is not always easy or even possible. But, on the other hand, nature will eventually heal even the worst cases, requiring, it is true, a longer time, and leaving behind very sad traces of her faulty workmanship. So that in treating a fracture, all these elements should be taken into consideration.

Fracture of the ribs: Bathe the swelling with THE MARVEL, and the parts will soon unite. Bandaging is of no consequence.

Fracture of the haunch-bone, cannot be reduced, but nature will ere long heal it, though with some distortion, one hip will be lower than the other

Fractures of the leg, from the weight of the animal, are extremely difficult to manage. It can only be done by suspending the animal by stout canvas passing under the belly and attached to rollers on either side, and by means of pulleys raising him up so that the feet just touch the ground, the canvas being supplied with heavy bands before and behind, to keep the body securely fixed in the canvas. The fractured ends of the limb should then be carefully adjusted, and the limb wound well with a roller-bandage, then a pair of iron splints, grooved so as to fit the limb, and well wadded with tow; the splint that is behind two or three inches longer than the foot, should be securely bound on. The whole internal bandage should be bathed in THE MARVEL, and kept wet with it, from time to time, for a week. This will subdue the inflammation, and hasten the union of the parts. After eight days, the splints should be removed and the limb examined, and again replaced, to remain five or six weeks, at the end of which time the splint may be removed, and a simple bandage and lighter splint retained until the cure is perfected in some six weeks longer, when the animal may be trusted to use his limb. If the ends are in proper apposition, and maintained there, the union will be perfect, with but little swelling or deformity.

The general treatment of all fractures is to place the parts in apposition, keep them there by proper splints and bandage, and keep the place wet with the MARVEL, until the heat and swelling have subsided. A dose of the Specific, B B, for SPRAINS and INJURIES, ten drops will be appropriate morning and night.

Luxation of the Patella, or Stifle.

Under the influence of a severe blow, a sudden leap or strain, the patella, or knee-pan is sometimes displaced. The animal holds his leg stiff and extended, cannot rest on it, and when obliged to walk, draws it along. This displacement of the patella is called being STIFLED. The displacement can be reduced by the aid of sufficient help, and placing a side-line with a hopple on the pastern of the affected limb, and, drawing the hind-leg forward, the surgeon will then, with both hands, bring the bone to its place.

Often the reduction is effected of itself if the horse makes the slightest effort. The part should be bathed in ARNICA or THE MARVEL, as the ligaments are always injured, and fifteen drops of the Specific, B B, for INJURIES, should be given three times per day.

Injuries of the stifle, bruises strains, etc., often occur, and should be treated by bathing the part with THE MARVEL or ARNICA, and giving the animal the above Specific for injuries.

Sprains and Dislocations.

Sprains of various joints or parts occur, which are more or less grave or serious. depending upon the extent of the injury or the joint involved. If a bone is displaced it is termed a dislocation. The joint becomes painful, swelling soon ensues, and on comparing the joint with its fellow, we perceive the distortion; the limb is longer or shorter, and the animal moves it with great difficulty or not at all. If the bone is not moved from its position, but the ligaments are merely injured, or torn, or joints otherwise bruised, it is termed a sprain. The swelling in this case is often as severe and even more so than in case of actual dislocation. Yet the accident is not so serious because in cases of horses and cattle, a dislocation is not always curable, and if the joint be replaced, the danger of new dislocation is far more imminent than though it had never occurred.

CAUSES.—Sprains and dislocations occur from false steps, slipping, leaping across ditches, sudden springing, violent effort in drawing a load, or sudden turning, or from falls, blows, kicks, contusions, etc.

TREATMENT —In all such cases the indications are simple, yet the execution of them sometimes very difficult. For sprains, bathe the parts with THE MARVEL, or ARNICA, to keep down the swelling and inflammation, renewing the application from time to time at intervals of two, four, or six hours, according to the urgency of the case, and give the Specific, B B, for INJURIES, two or three times a day until well; fifteen drops as a dose.

Sprains of the Fetlock.

A sprain of this joint sometimes occurs, manifested by heat, swelling, and lameness more or less decided, and especially manifested when the horse is moving on uneven ground. When recent, bathe the part with THE MARVEL, and saturate a bandage with it, and wrap it up moistening it from time to time, and giving the Specific, B B, for SPRAINS, two or three times per day, fifteen drops at a dose. The pain and lameness will gradually abate

Saddle-Galls, Galled Back or Breast.

Not unfrequently from long continued pressure of the saddle, or collar, or other portions of the harness, especially when not properly fitted, the part becomes injured or bruised. The result is a swelling of the part. Sometimes a small circular bruise or extravasation of blood, termed "warble," results, or these may ulcerate, producing in healing a thickening of the skin termed "sitfast." Thus we may have all grades from mere chafing and swelling to ulceration, cicatrization, and permanent scar.

TREATMENT.—In fresh injuries arising from chafing of the harness or saddle, apply THE MARVEL to the part two or three times per day, or if this is not at hand, ARNICA and cold water. A slight chafing or excoriation is relieved by cold water or salt and water.

Speedy Cut.

This term is applied to an injury on the enlargement of the splint bone inside of the leg immediately under the knee. A horse with high action in a fast trot violently strikes this part with the edge of the shoe or hoof.

SYMPTOMS.—This pain is often very great, so that horses have been known to drop like a shot; there is great heat and tenderness; more or less swelling and lameness. A bony enlargement is the result of repeated blows.

TREATMENT.—Give the horse rest or only such work as will prevent a repetition of the blow. Bathe the part with THE MARVEL, until the swel'ing is entirely reduced, or the swelling itself will cause a fresh injury. Alter the shoe so as to favor the interfering foot, draw it well under and rasp down the hoof as far as it will bear with safety, and see that the bearing is even all round. The inner side of the shoe should have but one nail, and that near the toe, if the work of the horse will admit of it.

Strains.

Strains of the tendons, or of different parts of an animal, occur, which are more or less serious according to circumstances, and which require medication for prompt and complete restoration.

A strain of the loins may occur from a leap off a bank, or from a slip, or from turning round in a stall. If severe, it is difficult to cure. The horse bends or lowers the quarters when walking, moves backward with difficulty, trots unsteadily, and thus refers his suffering to the loins. If very severe, he cannot move back or scarcely forward, drags his hind legs, and his quarters tremble when walking. In extreme cases he cannot raise himself, but sits on his haunches like a dog, soon falling again to the ground. There is heat, swelling, and tenderness of the lumbar region.

The shoulder may be strained by galloping on a hill side, or by a false slip in leaping, or by other effort causing a violent strain of the muscles of the shoulder. The suffering is quite severe, the animal is incapable of extending his shoulder, and therefore drags his toe on the ground in attempting to walk. The horse also goes down-hill with great difficulty. In some cases, there is considerable heat and swelling, and great pain when the shoulder is pinched. If the leg is lifted high up and drawn out forcibly forward, it causes great pain. This mark distinguishes the strain of the shoulder from any disease or lameness of the foot, that *it causes great pain to extend the limb forward, and, in standing, the horse places the leg before him not stretched out straight, but bent and resting on the toe.* After this condition of things has continued some time, a sinking in or depression is shown at the crest or top of the shoulder-blade, from inflammatory action and wasting of substance, to which the term SWENEY has been given.

Strain of the haunch, in which the animal halts a little, spares the affected limb as much as possible, and can neither trot or gallop When the strain is but slight, the animal scarcely limps in walking, and seems only pained when urged at a faster gait; when it is severe, even standing is painful, the animal limps in walking, and drags his leg; and in trotting, his buttocks describe a sort of swinging movement. It is often very difficult to detect it, but its presence may be inferred when a careful examination can discover no injury or lesion in any other part of the limb, and especially if the horse will not permit his haunch to be examined. It differs from spavin in that the lameness increases rather than diminishes by walking.

Strain of the tendons of the leg or of the enveloping sheath, is generally attended with excessive lameness and inflammation of the part, and the point of suffering is readily discovered.

TREATMENT.—In all cases bathe the part with the MARVEL or with ARNICA when the MARVEL is not to be had, and so long as there is heat, soreness, and swelling, continue to apply the wash every two or four hours. I prefer the MARVEL in all cases, yet the Arnica does very well The frequency of the application and length of time it should be continued, depends ou the extent or severity of the injury. Give also three times in the day, fifteen drops of the Specific for INJURIES, B B, according to the urgency of the symptoms. In old cases, a dose morning and night is sufficient; for more recent or fresh strains, a dose four times per day, until the more urgent symptoms are relieved.

In cases of strain of the shoulder or of the tendons, it is important to take the strain off the injured limb, and for this purpose a high shoe is best. Rivet two horse-shoes together two or three inches apart, the lower one the smallest, so as not to interfere in nailing, and keep this on until the strain is cured. Such a shoe is often necessary in many similar cases, to relieve the suffering or injured limb, by keeping the weight of the animal mainly upon the sound feet.

Stings of Bees, Hornets, &c.

Sometimes where a horse has been tied near a swarm of bees, if sweaty or otherwise offensive to them, the swarm has been known to attack and settle on him, producing pain, inflammation, and swelling, not unfrequently resulting in death. The stings of hornets are as bad or worse. The MARVEL applied freely, will relieve at once. Give at the same time the FEVER SPECIFIC A A, internally, fifteen drops, and repeat it every hour. If you have not the MARVEL use ARNICA in the same manner.*

Varices.

The veins of the leg are sometimes distended, especially at the point where the large vein passes over the inner surface of the hock joint, producing a soft elastic tumor. Bathe it with MARVEL, and give the remedy for INJURIES, B B, fifteen drops, morning and night.

Wounds.

Wounds differ much in importance and in the manner of treatment. Mere bruises or contusions only require the application of THE MARVEL or ARNICA, as before advised. Cuts made by a sharp instrument unite readily by bringing the parts neatly together and retaining them in place by adhesive plaster, or a few stitches. Those made by a ragged instrument require the same management, but often result in suppuration. Stab wounds are often most

* URTICA URENS (Stinging Nettle), or the PLANTAGO MAJOR—common 'ow plantain—are both valuable, if the former are not at hand. Make a strong tincture by bruising the leaves and stems of the PLANTAGO, then place it in a bottle or jar and, cover it with alcohol or even whiskey, and stir it well; it will be fit to apply in a few moments, and will promptly relieve. Of course, it improves with standing, and is efficient for stings of insects, bites of spiders, musquitoes, or even of venomous reptiles, snakes, etc. The plantain may be found almost everywhere in close yards or fields, and is invaluable for these purposes.

dangerous, as internal organs may have been wounded, and it is better not to heal up the surface wound. Gun-shot wounds are similar, and you can do but little for them. Extract the ball or shot if possible, and it will eventually heal of itself. When the belly has been ripped up, and the bowels protrude, it should be washed with tepid water, and examined carefully to see if it has been injured, and then replaced and the wound closed. If the bowel has been injured, and the animal can be used for the table it had best be killed at once.

When an artery has been wounded, the blood spurts out in jets and is very red; when a vein is injured the blood flows in an uniform stream, and is darker colored. Arterial wounds are far more dangerous, and the flow should be arrested promptly, either by compression or tying the artery itself. The application of THE MARVEL tends much to arrest the flow of blood. It is one of the best styptics known.

Very extensive wounds are soon followed by fever and inflammation commencing with a chill and the fever continuing several days. In some cases, after suppuration, unhealthy granulations, in the form of pale excrescences, arise from the bottom, which show no disposition to heal. THE MARVEL OF HEALING should be applied a few times to such unhealthy sores, until they assume a better color and appearance.

On stitching up a wound take the stitch from the inside, half an inch from the edge of the lip, bring the two edges together, and tie each stitch by itself, using as many as are required to keep the edges in place, and moisten the whole with the MARVEL to keep down the inflammation.

In cases where fever and inflammation ensue, a few doses of the Specific A A, for FEVER are of advantage, after which give the Specific B B, for INJURIES, fifteen drops three times per day.

If hemorrhage is very severe, lint soaked in the MARVEL, introduced into the wound, will soon arrest it.

When the knee or other joint has been penetrated by a wound, first cleanse it carefully from dirt and put on a compress saturated in the MARVEL, and bind it on with a long roller-bandage several yards in length, so as to keep it firm in place, and saturate it with the MARVEL from day to day. Should you not succeed in closing the wound, and thus arresting the flow of synovia, a hot iron may be used a little way around the joint, and the MARVEL compress again applied as before, taking care to tie the horse's head so as to keep him from disturbing the bandages. The operation may be repeated, if needful.

For injuries of the mouth apply the MARVEL, or a weak solution of ARNICA freely.

Wounds of the eye require to be bathed from time to time with the MARVEL, diluted one-half with water, and to give the Specific A A, for INFLAMMATION, ten drops three times per day, until the inflammation and swelling is subdued

In absence of the MARVEL, put two drops of the FEVER Specific in a glass of water and bathe the eye from time to time with it.

CHAPTER III.

DISEASES OF THE EYES, BRAIN, AND NERVES.

Albugo, or Spot in the Eye, Opacity of the Cornea.

In consequence of a blow, stroke of a whip, or similar injury, an inflammatory action is set up in the eye, the result of which is an effusion of serum between the lamina of the outer coating of the eye, which renders the cornea or clear part of the eye, whitish or opaque in spots, interfering materially with the sight and usefulness of the organ. But little can be done to remove those of long standing, but recent cases, or those where inflammation is just subsiding and the opacity only forming, will be dispelled by frequently bathing the eye with the MARVEL, and giving the Specific, A A, for INFLAMMATION, fifteen drops three times per day. In many cases of opacity a portion of soft honey, the size of a small pea, put in the eye daily, has been known to have a wonderful effect in removing such opacities.

Amaurosis, Gutta Serena.

This disease consists in entire or partial loss of vision in consequence of paralysis of the optic nerve, or interruption of its communication with the brain. Injuries of the head, or ball of the eye, or some disease of the brain, are the usual causes. The horse walks cautiously, head elevated, and ears move quickly backwards and forwards, the eye has a peculiar glassy appearance, and the pupil does not dilate and contract when light is brought near or removed from the eye.

But little can be done for these cases. In the earlier stages a dose of the Specific, A A, for INFLAMMATION, may possibly arrest its progress, but generally it is incurable in man or beast.

Cataract.

In consequence of injuries to the eye, blows, contusions, etc., or as a consequence of severe and repeated inflammation, the crystalline lens becomes opaque, so as to interfere with or altogether destroy the sight. On examining the eye, deep in the pupil a whitish, yellowish, or brownish body is discoverable. Sometimes, especially in the commencement, white streaks run from the centre outward, or the whole chamber within the pupil looks dim and whitish.

Old Cataracts are incurable, but recent and forming cases may be benefited by giving the Specific, A A, for INFLAMMATION, and that for INJURIES, B B, a dose (fifteen drops) every night alternately.

Ophthalmia, Inflammation of the Eye.

There are in the horse two well marked forms of Sore or Inflamed Eyes. ACUTE OPHTHALMIA and PERIODIC OR MOON BLINDNESS Acute inflammation occurs usually in consequence of some irritating substance, hay-seed, dust, etc., having got into the eye, or from overheating, heated food, or from hereditary predisposition.

SYMPTONS.—It comes on with heat and uneasiness, the animal keeps the eye closed, or dreads the light, the eye-ball and inside of the lid look red, and the ball is protruded and the eye secretes a quantity of water which runs down on the cheek, or of humour, which becomes purulent, and glues the lids together. The cornea is dim and whitish, or covered with a scum, the haw is swollen and red.

TREATMENT.—Examine the eye for dirt, hay-seed. hair, or other substances, and if found, carefully remove them. They are more frequently under the upper lid, which may be turned inside out over the point of the finger, by taking the lashes between the finger and thumb, and turning the lid upward. The eye should be bathed with the MARVEL, diluted one-half with water. or if this be not at hand, make a lotion. by putting four or five drops of the Specific for INFLAMMATION, A A, in a half-pint of pure, soft water, and the eye should be bathed with this two or three times per day, so long as the heat and swelling exist Give at the same time, in recent cases, fifteen drops of the FEVER SPECIFIC, A A, four times per day and in old cases the same dose morning and night. Arnica is of little consequence except where the inflammation is the result of a bruise.

PERIODIC OPHTHALMIA is really a general affection, the result of teething, and usually appears on the cutting of the middle incisors, the molars, and tusks, and hence, at the age of from three to five years.

SYMPTOMS.—Generally only one eye is attacked; the eye looks smaller, swims in tears, and is sensitive to the light, the cornea becomes dim and leaden, and the lens look gray. The pulse is full and freqent; the mouth hot, tongue dry, the water scanty and bowels constipated: There is evidently feverish excitement of the system and congestion of the blood to the head. Not unfrequently the inflammation passes from one eye to the other. Severe or repeated attacks are very apt to return again or leave as results, dimness of the cornea, opacity of the lens or cataract behind them..

TREATMENT.—Exclude the animal from the glare of the light, and give at once the Specific A A. for INFLAMMATION, ten drops every four or six hours. Bathe the eye from time to time with THE MARVEL, diluted with an equal quantity of soft water, or with the lotion mentioned in the case of Acute Ophthalmia. Keep him on low diet and the case will generally be soon relieved. As the eye improves, the intervals between the doses of medicine should be prolonged. Often a dose night and morning is sufficient. Given early it will prevent the development of serious consequences.

The Haw.

We mention in this connection a curious mechanism of the eye more to guard against abuses than to cure disease. Concealed within the inner corner of the eye, the margin only visible, is a black or pied triangular-shapen cartillage called the HAW, with its broad part forward. It is concave, exactly to suit the globe of the eye, and convex without, so as to adapt itself to the mucous lining of the lid, and the base of it is reduced to a thin, sharp edge. At the will of the animal this is rapidly protruded from its hiding-place, and passing swiftly over the eye, shovels up every nuisance mixed with tears, and then being suddenly drawn back, the dust or insect is wiped away as the haw again passes under the corner of the eye. The haw is subject in common with other parts of the eye to inflammation and swelling, and senseless grooms term this "the HOOKS," and have been known to draw the haw out and cut it off, to the lasting injury of the organ.

Such an inflammation only requires the usual treatment, and will be subdued by bathing the eye with THE MARVEL, diluted one half water, and giving the Specific for INFLAMMATION, A A, internally, ten drops as a dose and repeated morning and night.

Convulsions and Spasms, Apoplexy.

Occasionally, in consequence of high feeding and deficient exercise, and especially in fat young horses, with short necks and large blood-vessels, this disease occurs. It may also come on in consequence of drawing a heavy load up a hill, although in this case it is more likely to be a rupture of a blood-vessel, with hemorrhage from one or both nostrils. It is also predisposed by an overloaded stomach.

SYMPTOMS.—In apoplexy, the horse either suddenly falls down lifeless, or there are premonitory symptoms, such as vertigo, the animal holds his head down, or leans it upon something, yawns, perspires slightly, and moves clumsily, etc. Afterwards, the animal falls down suddenly, the circulation becomes disturbed and irregular, eyes red, protruded, and staring; breathing labored, short, rattling; body covered with sweat, and eyelids paralyzed. After a few convulsions the animal dies; or, in rare cases, an improvement takes place, to be again after a longer or shorter period of time, followed by relapse, or to result in paralysis. (Compare the symptoms with those of Epilepsy.)

TREATMENT.—So soon as any of the premonitory symptoms are observed, give at once the Specific for FEVER and CONGESTION, A A, fifteen drops, and repeat the dose every one, two, or three hours, until the animal is relieved, and then at longer intervals. If the horse falls under an attack of the disease give of the above Specific at once, and repeat the dose every half-hour or hour; remove the harness, etc., and from time to time pour some cold water upon the head, not too much or too violently, while you also give the medicine internally. Injections of salt and water also may be of decided advantage.

Epilepsy.

This disease sometimes appears in the horse, and manifests itself in the following manner: the animal suddenly trembles, remains standing for an instant with legs spread out, staggers. and then falls; convulsions ensue; he kicks, rolls, and twists himself about, grinds his teeth, passes his dung and urine involuntarily, froths at the mouth, the motions of the eye are spasmodic, irregular, and the respiration loud, painful, and sobbing. After a while he becomes quiet, breathing regular, and he gradually comes to himself as if coming out of a dream. The duration of a fit varies from a few minutes to several hours The attacks return again at periods varying from a few days to several weeks or months, generally coming at shorter intervals. Epilepsy differs from apoplexy as spasm differs from paralysis, and a little attention will not fail to distinguish them.

The causes are deep-seated changes in the nervous organism, and they are rarely curable.

TREATMENT.—Give, on any premonitions of an attack, the Specific for CONVULSIONS, A A, fifteen drops at once, and you will usually ward it off. For an attack, put a few drops in the mouth as soon as you can safely do it, and repeat it every half-hour or hour, until the paroxysm is ended. Afterwards, always give one dose to prevent a return. This treatment will sometimes avail.

Megrims, Fits, Vertigo, Congestion.

This is rather a frequent affection of the horse, and is a consequence of an undue pressure or rush of blood to the head, in most cases also excited by indigestion or over-fullness of the stomach.

In the milder cases, the horse stops suddenly, shakes his head or even staggers in evident giddiness and half-unconsciousness for a moment, and then goes on again as if nothing had happened. In more severe cases, he stops suddenly, shakes his head, falls or drops down, or after a few unconscious turns, and a violent struggle, will become insensible, and then rise up and go on again; such attacks closely simulate true epilepsy.

There are symptoms which indicate such an attack, and are plainly referable to congestion; such as dullness, indolence, dejection, the horse prefers the dark corner of the stable, his eyes are dull, look fixed and stupid, eyelids half shut, inattentive to everything, half asleep as it were, head hanging or resting on the manger. His gait is unsteady, heavy and slow, raises the feet high, and puts the entire sole to the ground, is awkward in turning, and can scarcely back at all. As the disease progresses, he becomes more and more insensible; mastication is performed slowly, dropping part from his mouth; prefers taking his food from the ground, and in drinking plunges his head into the water above his nostrils. Then there are violent moments, the animal runs on quite blind until some obstacle stops him; or he turns round, or remains tranquil, with head depressed and legs crowded beneath his body; without being able to change this unusual attitude, unless assisted to do so. The pulse is very slow, respiration slow, often sighing, tongue foul, mouth dry and clammy.

TREATMENT.—In all similar cases, whether incipient or fully developed, give first the Specific, A A, for CONGESTION, fifteen drops, and repeat it every one, two, or three hours, until the animal is relieved, or for twelve or twenty-four hours, and then at intervals of say four hours, alternate it with the Specific for INDIGESTION, J J, until restored. When this dozing, stupid condition mentioned above is present, indicating evident congestion to the head, fifteen drops of the Specific for CONGESTION A A, each morning and noon, and the same for INDIGESTION, J J, at night, will soon restore the animal again.

Paralysis.

Paralysis, entire or partial loss of nervous power over the muscles of certain parts or portions of the body, occasionally occurs in the horse as a consequence of mechanical injuries, severe cold, or some internal cause

When occuring in the face, the muscles of one side lose the power of motion; the lips hang down and seem swollen, are drawn to one side, or pulled upward; food is picked up and retained with difficulty, mastication is imperfect, and food drops readily from the mouth. Sometimes there is no feeling in the face or lips.

When the hinder part of the body is paralyzed, the horse is unable to rise or stand, sits on his haunches like a dog, and constipation and arrest of urination are very apt to be present. In slighter cases, the hind-legs sway about clumsily, or he drags them after him, or even walks on his fetlocks.

TREATMENT.—The first course, in case of recent paralysis, is to give the Specific for CONGESTION, A A, fifteen drops every two hours, which continue one day; then give the Specific, J J, for PARALYSIS, fifteen drops every four, or six hours, according to the circumstances, until relieved, and then morning and night for a time.

Inflammation of the Brain, Phrenitis, Mad Staggers.

This disease is most frequently met with in entire horses, and attacks especially those that are ardent, in high condition, but little worked; and it is liable to be excited by a chill after being over-heated or over-worked in hot weather. It may also arise from blows or similar injuries on the head.

SYMPTOMS.—In some cases it comes on slowly; the horse is dull and sleepy; rests his head on the manger, or places it against the wall or between his legs, and falls asleep. In this state he will, perhaps, stagger and almost fall to the ground; he, however, wakes up, stares about him, takes a mouthful of hay, chews it slowly, and ere long is again dozing or fast asleep. The eyelids are nearly closed; the eyes and nose red; the pupils dilated; the bowels bound, and pulse slower than in health. This is the congestive stage, and may continue until the animal recovers or dies; but, in general, other symptoms appear to which the name Mad Staggers may be more appropriately applied In such cases the pulse rises; the breathing is quickened; the nose and eyes are very red; nostrils widened; the eyes have a wild, fierce look; the feet are stamped, as if in passion; he plunges about the stall, rears upward, strikes out with his fore-feet, and falls backward upon the ground, where he lies panting and covered with sweat; his eyes are thrust forward out of their sockets, and rattles are heard in the throat. Towards the end these violent paroxysms are repeated from time to time, and it is very dangerous to approach or go near him. At last, he is so weak and prostrate that he can not rise, and amidst convulsions, strangling, foaming at the mouth, sweating, and panting for breath, the animal dies.

TREATMENT.—The treatment will not be difficult, or the result doubtful, during the congestive stage; but in the fully developed or phrentic stage, quite so in both respects. The Specific for INFLAMMATION and CONGESTION, A A, is the principal dependence, and a dose of fifteen drops may be given every two or three hours, at first, and as the horse improves, the intervals may be somewhat prolonged. Continue this treatment steadily and without deviation. During the paroxysms, the medicine may be given by means of a small glass syringe, or the Medicator used in a similar manner. After the more intense symptoms have passed over, some doses of the remedy for INDIGESTION, J J, alternately with that for INFLAMMATION, A A, will be of value, giving one in the morning, and the other at night.

Concussion of the brain, inducing symptoms and a condition not essentially varying from the above, requires the same treatment, together with such external applications as the wound may require.

Tetanus, or Lock-Jaw.

This disease is more common in the horse than in other domestic animals. It consists of a muscular spasm of the jaw (whence its name), which usually from thence extends to all the muscles of the body. It most frequently occurs in consequence of an injury or wound, such as broken knees, open joints, severe bruises, nicked or docked tail, castration, wounds of the feet, prick of a nail, or even the galling of a crupper. It is also caused by cold or damp, sudden arrest of strangles, worms, or a bad condition of the stomach

SYMPTOMS.—In general it comes on very slowly, but also, in some cases, with great violence. The muscles of the neck and jaw are first affected, so that the horse has great difficulty in swallowing and turning his neck. The muscles then become quite stiff; the mouth is nearly closed; the jaws cannot be parted, and little or no food can be taken into the mouth. By degrees all the muscles become affected with the same stiffness and cramp; the eyes are still and staring, pulled back into their sockets, and squinted outward, and the haw is thrust forward; the neck can not be bent and the muscles feel hard and firm, the head can not be raised or lowered, and is held forward, with the nose stretched out; the nostrils are expanded; the ears pointed forward, erect, and fixed; the lips are firmly stretched across the teeth, which are partly seen; the saliva flows from the mouth; and the horse looks anxious, and can scarcely move, the belly is hard and tucked up; the tail is lifted up and held straight out, and in constant tremble; the legs are firmly fixed to the ground, and spread out from each other; the bowels are bound, and urine passed with difficulty; the breathing is quickened, labored and convulsive; the pulse is disturbed easily by frightening or speaking angrily to the horse, and it becomes afterward weak and trembling. While the spasm of the muscles continue, the animal is in constant pain, although it is less severe at some times than others.

TREATMENT.—Where a wound or injury has taken place, and tetanus supervenes, it will be of course traced directly to this, and the wound should at once be treated as recommended for that particular case. If the discharge has suddenly stopped, it should be reproduced by mild, warm applications to the part, and any irritation of the wound allayed as soon and as far as possible.

The horse should also be treated with the greatest possible kindness, not to be handled roughly or unkindly, and as the spasms are rendered more intense or severe from fright or noise, the groom must not shout or speak angrily; everything must be done in the most kind and quiet manner, and no glare of light admitted into the stable for the same reason. The medicine can be given by the Medicator, thrown well back into the mouth.

So soon as any stiffness of the jaws, or other indication of this disease appears, give fifteen drops of the Specific, A A, for CONVULSIONS, and repeat the dose every three hours. Should an improvement not take place in twenty-four hours, whether occasioned by any injury or otherwise, alternate the Specific for PARALYSIS, J J, with the first-named, at intervals of three or four hours, and continue this treatment perseveringly. In some cases the Specific for PARALYSIS, J J, may be used to advantage from the first, but the two remedies will generally be found most successful in alternation.

When the disease has become fully developed, or appears very violent, or does not promptly yield to the remedies, we advise the following course, from a full conviction that, if perseveringly fo lowed the animal may be promptly saved. One case has been reported to me in which the recommendation was carried out with entire success After six buckets of cold water had been used the chill came on, with prompt relaxation of the spasm which never returned, and the animal made a prompt recovery.

Provide several buckets or tubs of water, as cold as it can be made, the colder the better, even if swimming in snow and ice, as the object is to reduce the temperature of the animal as rapidly as possible.

Provide conveniently also several blankets and parts of blankets or cloths, to wrap up the entire body, neck, and legs. These should be conveniently at hand, so as to envelop the animal as soon as possible after having been thoroughly chilled. Then standing the animal where the water will conveniently run off, proceed gently to pour the water over the animal from a pitcher, in a moderate stream. Two persons can do it best, each with pitchers, being constantly replenished from the buckets behind them, at the rate of a bucketful each in three or four minutes, pouring the stream from the top of the head, so on along down the neck and spine, constantly changing the direction of the streams and keeping them running over the animal, until he is *thoroughly chilled, through and through, and shakes and trembles violently.* This is the criterion, and the streams must be kept up until this is accomplished, whether it requires twenty minutes or two hours, or longer.

As soon as this is accomplished, and the horse *shakes and trembles violently,* remove him to a comfortable place, wipe off the superfluous water, and wrap him in blankets from head to heels, enveloping the neck and muzzle, body and limbs, in several folds, pinning them closely and throwing an extra one, or buffalo-robe, over the whole, to invite the return of warmth and perspiration. Usually, and if the animal has been thoroughly chilled, with return of warmth, perspiration will break out all over him, and the disease is gone. If the animal has not been sufficiently chilled, only a dry heat will come on, and the spasms remain. The operation must then be repeated, until the result is obtained. But if the animal be thoroughly chilled and treated as above, a warm perspiration will come on, with entire relief of the spasm.

The horse will then be well, and only need careful and gradual removal of the superfluous covering, so as not to chill the animal again or permit him to take cold.

During this entire process the medical treatment, as above mentioned, must be continued, and for some time after, to prevent a return.

FOOD.—When the jaws are firmly set, no food can be given, but there are times when the spasms relax, and the jaws are rather wider than at other periods. Green food and gruel may then be offered to the horse. When the jaws becomes more open, he may have bran, clover, or hay-tea, gruel, and such similar food. If the jaws can not be opened, or he can not swallow, meal or oatmeal-gruel may be injected, by means of a large syringe, into the fundament, and life be thus prolonged.

Care must be taken to feed sparingly when recovering, or indigestion and a fatal result may be the consequence.

CHAPTER IV.

DISEASES OF THE NOSE AND AIR-PASSAGES.

Chill.

This term is used to designate a transitory state or condition, which may either terminate in recovery, or in severe inflammatory disease of some important organ or affection, of which the chill is the first stage. When a chill is present it is impossible to say, with certainty, whether or what further derangement will ensue But it is quite certain an abnormal condition is already present, with the probability that it will develop some disease or inflammation, of which we now have the first or forming stage. Usually the length and violence of the chill is in proportion to the importance of the organ attacked, and the character of the morbid influence.

The *direct* causes of a chill are: exposing the animal to cold draughts; allowing him to drink freely of cold water, in very hot or during very cold weather; exhausting him with labor and then placinghim in a damp stable; washing the legs with cold water, or riding him (while in a state of perspiration), into a stream of cold water.

SYMPTOMS.—The symptoms which are usually observed before the chill proper sets in, are: dullness or want of spirit on entering a stable after a journey: hanging of the head; standing fixedly in one place; taking little or no notice when spoken to; smelling at the food; picking amongst it for a short time and then leaving it altogether.. In addition to these, the eye is dull and countenance dejected; the animal grinds his teeth and breathes quicker than usual, while the pulse is rarely or never disturbed at the commencement. Soon the coat will begin to prick and the animal will begin to tremble with considerable violence; his breathing will become more hurried, attended with a harsh blowing sound in the nasal passages; the pulse still retaining its usual slow beat. Sometimes the breathing becomes quick, hurried, and loud · "panting." This condition may continue half an hour, or even two hours or more, when the patient will become more quiet, the breathing softer, more tranquil, the skin and extremities warmer, and the pulse rises to fifty or even sixty beats to the minute. From this condition the attack may, under judicious treatment, pass off, and speedy recovery ensue; or, it may pass into a Catarrhal Fever, or Pneumonia, or Bronchitis, or Lymphitis, or Laminitis, or Inflammation of the Bowels, or what is quite common, a bad, obstinate cough.

TREATMENT.—With as little delay as may be, the patient should be comfortably housed and blanketed, and fifteen drops of the SPECIFIC A A, for INFLAMMATION, should be given. If not better in half an hour, repeat it, and again at intervals of half an hour, until the trembling and respiration have been relieved and the chill has passed off. Then the animal may be safely left under the influence of the same medicine, to be repeated every two or three hours, so long as circumstances seem to require it.

Should any of the diseases above mentioned or other, have become developed, the treatment must be varied to meet that condition; the particulars of which are to be sought under the respective sections in this MANUAL. But it will most frequently be found that having met and conquered the enemy at the threshold, but little more remains to be done beyond care and rest, for the entire recovery of the patient.

Catarrh or Cold, Influenza, Catarrhal Fever, Epidemic Catarrh.

THE nose and air-passages are lined with a delicate membrane, whose office it is to secrete a thin mucus which lubricates the parts. Under the influence of a chill, suppressed perspiration, etc., this membrane becomes irritated, inflamed, and the discharge arrested, or it is thickened, increased, or variously modified.

The SYMPTOMS usually are, the horse is not so lively as usual; he eats little or no food; he coughs and sneezes; a watery discharge flows from one or both nostrils, and also from the eyes, which are red and swelled.

In the more severe form, there is a chill, warm skin, quick pulse, frequent and somewhat difficult breathing, sore throat, pain in the throat when pinched, frequent cough, rough coat, bound bowels, red eyes, and red and dry nose; tears flow freely, and little or no food is eaten—all symptoms indicating a catarrhal fever. As the animal improves, the discharge from the nose becomes white or yellowish, and more profuse.

Where numerous horses are attacked about the same time, the symptoms assume a more severe form, attended with a greater degree of prostration than in cases of common cold, and it then merits the name of INFLUENZA. The symptoms of one year vary from those of another, and during the same season all animals are not handled alike, though the general outline will be the same. The attending fever is of a low grade, comes on suddenly, and soon reaches its height, and lowness of spirits and weakness are predominant. The symptoms are often as follows:

The horse is dull, low-spirited, and easily tired; he yawns and hangs his head; his coat stares; sweats easily, and breathes quickly, when slightly worked or moved. He eats little or nothing. As the disease advances, the skin is sometimes hot and again cold; the mouth and tongue are dry and hot; the white of the eye and nose are red; the bowels bound; urine scanty; the eyelids swelled, partly closed, tears flow down the face and fret the skin. The sides of the nostrils are also fretted by the acrid discharge from them, which is sometimes very profuse. The throat is so much inflamed that swallowing is attended with pain and difficulty—the animal "quids" his food, and splashes the water with his muzzle, being afraid to swallow either fluid or solid food. The throat is painful, hot, and swelled on the outside; the glands are also swelled, hard, and painful, and sometimes maturate. The cough is frequent, sometimes coming on in fits, and breathing is sometimes quite obstructed and difficult. When the disease has lasted some time, the dung is slimy and mixed with blood, and the discharge from the nose is sometimes bloody.

A common cold may terminate in inflammation of the bronchia or lungs, by extending downwards, or it may be cured and expend itself merely in the nose and throat. So an Influenza may extend and involve the pulmonary tissue, and is far more grave than is usually supposed.

TREATMENT.—When the disease commences with a chill, or any considerable degree of Fever is present, give fifteen drops of the SPECIFIC for FEVER, A A, and repeat it several times, at intervals of two or three hours. Then alternate the SPECIFIC for COUGH E E, with the Fever medicine, at intervals of three or four hours, until the disease is broken up and the horse is well. In case of Influenza, even with very threatening symptoms, the SPECIFIC, for COUGH, E E, and for FEVER, A A, should be given alternately, say every four hours, in doses of fifteen drops; keeping the animal well covered and in a warm stable. After all the feverish symptoms have disappeared, only the COUGH SPECIFIC, E E, will be required, and the intervals between the doses may be prolonged as the animal improves. In case the discharge from the nose is profuse or thick, and excoriating, or when the sore throat is present, or predominates, one or both of the above-mentioned remedies may be omitted, and the SPECIFIC for DISTEMPER, C C, be given instead, at the same intervals, and doses, and this may be continued to the conclusion of the case, either alone or in alternation with the Specific E E, for COUGH.

Canadian Horse Disease.

This disease made its appearance in the Canadas, in the winter, or early spring of 1872, and gradually, but sometimes with rapid strides, extended southward along the great lines of travel, attacking successfully a very large proportion of all the horses in Toronto and the larger towns of Canada; then in Buffalo and in Rochester, and thence in New York, Boston, Providence, Albany, Troy, thence southward to Philadelphia, Baltimore, Washington, and so extending southward and westward over the entire country. Answering the laws which govern all great epidemics among men, it extended in succession over all our large cities, and involved with a greater or lesser degree of severity, the entire open country, subjecting to its influence almost every horse within its range.

The immediate fatality was not great, yet almost every horse was affected, and with few rare exceptions, all laid up for several days, while in numerous cases fatal termination occurred from want of care, work during the attack, exposure, and from the violence of the disease in old worn out animals, or those predisposed to lung diseases, or improper medical treatment.

Pure blood stock was less seriously affected than coarse animals, and the disease was much more serious and fatal among the latter.

The disease is essentially a Catarrhal Fever, of an epizootic nature, the result of some atmospheric influence, as is shown by its sudden appearance over a large extent of country, attacking with but slight discrimination all kinds of horses, old and young, and those in good condition as well as the poor or enfeebled.

The premonitory symptoms are: Dullness, low spirits, hanging the head, easily fatigued, and sweats on exercise, a staring coat, a *watery discharge from the nose*, speedily followed by a severe hacking Cough; or the warning cough precedes all other symptoms a day or two. The pulse becomes quickened, and the mouth hot; the nasal mucus membrane becomes injected and red, pinkish, or even lead color, and the ears and legs unnaturally cold. Gradually the discharge from the nose increases, and becomes of a greenish yellow color, and as the disease extends along the mucus surface, the throat becomes sore, the glands involved, and the swallowing impeded painful and difficult, and as the bronchia becomes involved, the respiration is increased in frequency, and in some cases becomes labored and difficult.

In the progress of the disease, the glands may

become swelled, and even suppurate, the throat filled with superficial ulcerations, resulting in profuse and debilitating discharges from the nose, or the disease process may involve the entire larynx, bronchia, and even pulmonary tissue, giving rise to difficult, oppressed breathing, imperfect æration of blood, and other results of pneumonia.

As the disease yields, the temperature of the patient becomes more uniform, the pulse and heat lowered, the breathing more free, the discharge thicker and diminished in quantity, the sore throat yields, and appetite and general condition improve until convalescence is established.

PREVENTIVE TREATMENT

You may, by taking more than usual care of the animals during the prevalence of an epizooty, and before the symptoms declare themselves, *prevent* the access of the disease by giving fifteen drops of the SPECIFIC, C C, for DISTEMPER, every morning and night, during its prevalence. If the attack is not fully prevented, it may be so modified as to be of but slight consequence and readily controlled.

TREATMENT DURING THE DISEASE.

With the first symptoms of the disease Dullness, staring coat, *watery discharge from the nose*, slight occasional or even severe cough:—commence by giving fifteen drops of SPECIFIC C C, which may be repeated every three hours during the day, giving a dose late at night, and then, unless the animal is very sick, it may be omitted until the early morning, when it should be resumed, and so continued from day to day. As the disease yields, or the animal improves, the medicine requires to be given less frequently, and the doses may be given at intervals of four and six hours.

Should the disease be more advanced, and especially should there be *fever* manifested by a chill, heat of the mouth or surface, increased frequency of pulse and respiration, severe frequent cough, even should the ears and legs be unnaturally cool or cold, the SPECIFIC A A, should be given at intervals of three hours, alternately with the C C; that is fifteen drops of A A, should be given, and after three hours fifteen drops of C C, and so on in alternation at intervals of three hours This alternation of remedies should be continued until the circulation is equalized, the cough and respiration relieved, and a general improvement manifest, when the A A may be omitted and the C C continued at intervals of four or six hours until the cure is complete.

Should the secretions from the nose become diminished, or dried up with *increased difficulty of breathing*, which is evidently painful and labored, showing the development of Pneumonia from the extension of the disease to the lungs, the SPECIFIC E E for COUGHS, will be required, and may be given a dose of fifteen drops every three hours, giving it alone; or, if there is yet considerable heat or fever, it may be given in alternation with the FEVER

SPECIFIC A A until the fever is allayed, when the A A may be discontinued and cure perfected by the use of the E E.

IF THE COUGH is not troublesome, but the discharge from the head becomes very profuse like a nasal gleet or even the glanders, the SPECIFIC C C, is only required, and may be given in doses of fifteen drops four times per day, and continued until the cure is perfected. See also the section on Glanders and Nasal gleet.

If the legs, sheath, lips or nose swells, or decided dropsy sets in, give the SPECIFIC H H, alternately with the C C, fifteen drops every two or three hours, in alternation, which continue until relieved.

For the weakness, dullness, or loss of appetite which may remain after the acute attack has passed over, give fifteen drops of the SPECIFIC J J for INDIGESTION three times per day. It will promptly improve the appetite and give tone and strength to the system.

NURSING AND CARE DURING TREATMENT.

The animal should be excused from all service, and allowed complete rest. The stables should be clean and well ventilated, and free from any noxious accumulations or exhalations. Lime, Chloride of Lime or White-wash, may be freely employed, but the use of penetrating so-called disinfectants is not admissible under Homeopathic treatment. The patient should be properly groomed, and the nose and mouth frequently sponged, being careful not to communicate the discharge from the nose to the eyes. Better keep a separate sponge for the eyes. The horse should be comfortably blanketed, and if the legs are cold, they should be bandaged. The drink may have the chill slightly removed, but not made so warm as to be unpalatable. The diet should be light, and of a laxative nature. Bran, or spout feed wet with warm water, or made up in a mash, with a little salt added. Gruels, of meal, oat-meal, mixed with bran or midlins, with a little salt, are best, especially during the height of the disease and prevailing sore throat. Carrots, or similar green food and hay, in moderate quantities, are allowable.

Exercise in mild genial weather may be allowed, if the force of the disease has passed, or when it is but slight from the first, and in very mild cases, occasional use may be allowed.

Most animals are sick from five to fifteen days—mismanaged or neglected cases for a much longer period, while some cases run into after diseases which ultimately prove fatal.

Spinal Meningitis.

This disease has become quite common in late years, sometimes appearing in isolated cases, but more frequently prevailing in certain cities or sections of country; and to such an extent as to warrant the idea of an epidemic influence. Often a large number of horses in a city, or quite a proportion of those working a city railroad, are more or less seriously attacked. It is mostly observed in the winter and spring, and is favored by changeable weather, damp or too close stables; appears more requently on horse railroad and stage lines, from he frequent sudden stops, and severe strain of the loins in starting It is also more common among mares, from their being overworked or strained when in heat.

THE EARLIER SYMPTOMS ARE: Dullness, indisposition to move, head hanging low, and evident pain and stiffness on moving, and especially on being turned around There is more or less tenderness, and shrinking on pressure on some portion of the spine or along the entire spine, from the hips forward, or on each side over the kidneys. The animal does not stand or move firmly, but sways from side to side in walking; or is easily pushed one side, or even over, when standing. Finally the back gives out, and the horse falls down, or cannot rise; he has no strength in the hind legs The pulse at first is not much, or but slightly increased in frequency or force, but by degrees becomes more rapid. The urine is often scanty or suppressed, and the dung dry, and the animal has from the first a distressed, suffering look.

The disease is frequently fatal, in the more severe cases, in two or three days, but often continues from seven to ten days, and recoveries are usually quite slow.

TREATMENT.—From the first, the principal remedy is the SPECIFIC A A. This should be given in doses of fifteen drops at first, every hour; then after six or eight hours—the intervals may be every two hours, and as the animal improves, the intervals between doses may be prolonged to three or even four hours.

If, during the disease, THE URINE, or staling, should become *very scanty*, or be passed *with difficulty*, or *with straining*, or BE SUPPRESSED, then the Specific H H, for urinary or kidney affections, will be in place, and it should be given a dose of fifteen drops in alternation with the A. A. That is, give the A A, and after two hours give the H. H, then after two hours, again give the A A, and so giving the two in alternation, until the secretion of water is fully established, when the use of the H H, may be discontinued.

AFTER THE MORE URGENT STAGE OF THE DISEASE HAS PASSED OVER, the heat and fever mostly gone, and there yet remains SOME WEAKNESS, OR PARTIAL PARALYSIS OF THE LOINS, indicated by inability to rise, swaying, tottering, or shambling gait, the specific J J, is the remedy, and it may be given in the same doses, fifteen drops, either in alternation with A A, if feverish symptoms yet remain, or alone, at intervals of four or six hours, to complete the cure. It is the special remedy for partial or complete paralysis, or for the weakness and debility remaining after sickness.

The horse should have a loose box, or wide, roomy stall well littered and reasonably warm, and in cool or cold weather, be well covered with blankets, and his legs should be occasionally well hand-rubbed. Let him have bran mashes, or carrot tea, and pick at some good hay. The animal should not be exercised or worked too soon after recovery, for fear of a relapse.

Pink Eye.

This disease is well known among horse dealers, and in the stables of all our large cities. It is not so often found in the open country, but cases occur where green or young horses are taken from pasture and subjected to the closer atmosphere and changed diet of a warm stable. It is generally found among green horses who have been brought from the country to our large cities for sale or use, and quite a large proportion of all such horses are, more or less seriously affected by it. The disease is really a Catarrhal Influenza, whose symptoms are variously modified and only possibly received the now generally accepted name of PINK EYE, from a frequent appearance of the eye in the earlier stages of the malady. The supposed causes have been sufficiently above hinted.

SYMPTOMS.—There is a wide diversity in the symptoms, but the more common manifestations are as follows ; The horse is first observed to be *dumpish*, dull, and disinclined to move, or moving clumsily, and looks as if he had been sick; the vessels of the eye are distended, turgid, the inner lid and corners being unnaturally red, (whence probably, the name), the lids become swollen, the animal shrinks from the light and tears trickle over the eyelid, and lumps of purulent matter occasionly gum up or fill the angles. The head seems heavy and hangs down, or he rests it upon the manger. First one hind leg and then the other swells and becomes infiltrated with fluid, extending from the fetlock up and filling the sheath, and often along under the belly with an immense infiltration of fluid. This swelling is considered characteristic, comes on suddenly, affects the whole limb, groin and sheath. The hair from the first looks unhealthy and has a rough feeling; the ears, nose, and limbs are cold or wet, according to the stage of the disease. The appetite is poor from the first, and an attempt to swallow shows that the throat is sore; the fauces will be found inflamed, the tongue is foul, thickly coated, and saliva runs freely, though in some cases the mouth is dry and feverish; the dung is voided in small quantities, as all the functions seem torpid In some cases the glands of the neck become involved, tenderness and swelling is found on examination, and this swelling may soften and terminate in an abscess under the jaw. There is not unfrequently a cough. After a few days, a discharge from the nose sets in, which is considered a favorable crisis.

TREATMENT.—The patient should have the benefit of a pure atmosphere—the more elevated, pure, and uncontaminated, the better to arrest blood deterioration—and be covered according to the temperature of the stable and season. The limbs may be rubbed and clothed if cold, but not rubbed if they are hot and feverish. In the febrile stage the natural covering is sufficient Fat horses need but trifling food, and bran mashes, scalded spout feed, or green food in moderation are best until the turn of the disease.

Give with the first indication of the disease, the SPECIFIC A A, for INFLAMMATION, which repeat at intervals of three hours, in doses of fifteen drops. This may be continued one, two or more days, so long as the pulse is quick, mouth hot, or general fever, or swelled reddish eyes. When, however, *the throat* is found to be sore, *glands* under the jaws *swelled or tender* on pressure, or there is a discharge from the nose, the SPECIFIC C C for DISTEMPER, is more appropriate, and should be substituted for the A A, and be given at the same doses and intervals. If, however, there is yet with the above, fever and heat, the two Specifics may be given alternately—first A A, then C C, at intervals of three hours between the doses.

After the *legs* and *sheath* have begun to swell, the SPECIFIC H H for DROPSY is in order, and should be given to rouse into activity the urinary secretion, and so reduce the swelling. Give then the SPECIFIC H H, every three hours, in alternation with the C C, and so continue until the disease is arrested and the patient is convalescent. Too great care cannot be exercised when the legs are swelled, to *let the horse stand*, not to move or exercise the patient, as the movement or exercise while the legs are swelled or hot, invariably aggravates the difficulty, and may cause it to extend to the lungs or other important organs. Take the feed away, or keep the feed very low, no grain, only a bran-mash, or pick at a little hay, and let the horse stand, and the swelling will disappear with the use of the medicines mentioned, H H. If from cold or exposure, or an extension of the morbid process, the *lungs should become involved* and Pneumonia be present, the disease will require to be treated by the SPECIFICS A A, and E E, as directed for that disease, which see.

Any weakness, or loss of appetite or condition, remaining as a sequel of the disease, will be removed by the use of SPECIFIC J J, giving fifteen drops three times a day.

Cough.

Cough is so well known as to require no description It is in almost all cases a mere symptom of some disease or morbid condition of the air passages, such as a cold, bronchitis, catarrh, or other more serious affection of the chest, upon the cure of which it disappears. In some cases, however, this affection is so slight as to occasion only cough as a symptom of its existence, and the cough may be said to be idiopathic. Continued cough predisposes to inflammation, yet some horses have a slight cough for years without being otherwise unwell. Other coughs are connected with thick wind, broken wind, glanders, worms, and indigestion.

TREATMENT.—For all chronic coughs fifteen drops of the SPECIFIC for COUGHS, E E, morning and night, are sufficient. In more complicated or recent cases, the medicine may be given three or four times per day. Sometimes the SPECIFIC A A, for INFLAMMATION, is equally or more efficient, even when no fever or heat is apparent.

Spasms of the Diaphragm or Midriff

This is a very rare disease in the horse, but may occur in consequence of disorders of the stomach and bowels, or violent exertions when the stomach is distended with food.

SYMPTOMS.—The midriff contracts with so much force that the whole body is shaken and a "thumping" noise is heard at some distance; these thumps are best heard when the ear is placed over the back at each side of the spine; the pulse is small, from fifty to sixty to the minute, and the breathing from twenty to thirty; the breath is drawn quickly into the lungs, and is attended with a sniffling sound at the nose; the sides of the nose are drawn inward, when the breath is inhaled

This thumping or spasm differs from palpitation of the heart by the number of beats being different from that of the heart, by the sounds being heard over the back and the drawing in of the nostrils during inspiration.

TREATMENT.—The disease will be cured by giving the SPECIFIC for FEVER, A A, or by giving the FEVER and COUGH SPECIFIC, E E, alternately, fifteen drops every three hours.

Heaves, Broken Wind, Thick Wind, Whistles.

These are merely varieties of nearly one and the same pathological condition, and the distinctions lead to no practical result in my method of treatment.

THICK WIND is generally the result of an imperfectly cured bronchitis or pneumonia, leaving either the mucous membrane of the bronchia permanently thickened, or some portions of the lung more or less solidified, thus impairing its capacity and diminishing or destroying its elasticity. Hence, the horse when exercised especially up hill, breathes short, hurriedly, and more laboriously than in health. This causes much distress, the horse expands his nostrils, heaves, pants and breathes with difficulty.

BROKEN WIND is the result of *emphysema* of the lungs, that is, the minute air-cells in certain portions of the lungs become dilated, lose their elasticity or power of contraction, and breaking one into another, form variously-sized sacks of air, the entrance to which becomes closed, so that this air remains resident in the lungs and so far destroys its use. Spasm of the air-tubes acts in a similar manner, hence, it may come and go, but the former condition is more or less permanent. Spasm, or disease of the midriff, is frequently connected with it. The usual symptoms are, the flanks are slowly drawn up until they have a tucked-up appearance, when they suddenly fall down. The act of forcing the air *from the lungs* is far more difficult, and requires longer time than to *inspire* or draw it in. There is also a short, weak, wheezing cough, rough, dry coat; greediness for food, yet the animal is thin and looks poor; the belly is swelled with wind; oats often pass unchanged from the bowels.

TREATMENT —Some cases of broken and thick wind cannot be cured, as they depend upon organic changes in the structure of the lungs, themselves incurable, yet all can be benefited and many are entirely cured by the persistent use of the proper Specific remedies, and proper attention to food and work.

In all cases of this disease of whatever variety, if recent or extensive, give fifteen drops of the COUGH SPECIFIC, E E, noon and at night, and the same of the SPECIFIC A A, each morning. In old, long-standing cases, give fifteen drops of the Specific A A, every morning, and the same of Specific E E at night, continuing the treatment with perseverance.

FOOD —As the animal suffers from want of space in the chest, so the distension of the stomach with an undue quantity of food tends much to increase the difficulty. Hence the most condensed form of food is best, plenty of oats and little hay, but no chaff, straw, or bloating feed, water in moderate quantities, but never to repletion until the day's work is over. Green food, carrots especially, are always useful. They are readily digested, and are peculiarly beneficial to the respiratory organs. On the contrary, bloating, flatulent, poor feed, will tend to increase and may even occasion, broken wind. The horse should not be worked soon after a full meal.

Bronchitis.

From exposure to wet and cold; sudden changes of weather; turning the horse into a cold wet place or bringing him from grass to a warm stable; standing in a draft of cold air, or washing the warm sweating skin and not drying it afterwards, an inflammation of the bronchial tubes and minute air-cells takes place, meriting the name of BRONCHITIS.

SYMPTOMS.—The disease generally begins with a slight cough, quick breathing, sore throat, low spirits, dislike of food, slight discharge from the nostrils, pain of the throat when pinched, and some difficulty of swallowing. In some cases, it comes on suddenly with shaking; the legs, ears, and muzzle are at one time hot and at another cold; the skin is rough and staring; the head hung down; mouth hot; the animal remains standing, and does not wish to move; pulse is full and quick; the cough short, frequent, and irritating; the breathing quick and difficult: the eyes and nose red, and rattles are heard in the windpipe at the breast. A profuse discharge of matter from the nostrils indicates the period from which improvement commences.

TREATMENT.—Give the SPECIFIC for FEVER, A A, and that for COUGH, E E, fifteen drops alternately every three hours, beginning with Specific A A. After a day or two as the animal improves the intervals between the doses may be prolonged to four or six hours. Keep the animal well covered and protected until recovery takes place. After the feverish symptoms have disappeared, the COUGH SPECIFIC, E E, may be relied upon for the perfection of the cure, given three or four times per day.

STABLING AND FOOD.—In all cases of serious disease of the lungs or air-passages, the horse should be placed in a large roomy stable or stall into which the fresh air may freely come, but all damp draughts of air excluded; all dung, damp and dirty straw carefully removed; spread clean straw on the floor; blanket him according to the season, the state of the weather, and skin; hand-rub and flannel-bandage the legs every night and morning, or oftener if necessary.

For food, bran mashes, gruel, and tempered water only; when recovering, malt or bran mashes, boiled oats, turnips, carrots, and green food, if in season.

Inflammation of the Larynx. Laryngitis.

The larynx is the upper portion of the windpipe and inflammation of it sometimes occurs and is very dangerous It is not often unmixed, but is generally accompanied with, or is an extension of, cold or bronchitis, and its causes are the same.

It is sometimes a dangerous disease, and may kill by suffocation or degenerate into bronchitis or pneumonia. It is recognized by the difficulty of respiration, WHICH IS LOUD AND HEARD AT A DISTANCE.

The outside of the throat is hot, painful and swelled; swallowing is sometimes difficult, and the fluid even may return by the nose; the breathing is short and difficult, and when the air is drawn into the lungs a rough harsh sound is heard in the larynx; the cough, at first short and hard, becomes more hoarse and feeble, and occurs in fits especially during an attempt to swallow; the pulse is quick, hard and full, and skin hot As the disease advances, the breathing becomes more difficult, and is attended with a rasping, crowing sound, the neck is straightened and held stiffly, the head raised and larynx drawn towards the breast, the nostrils are widened, the nose lead colored, the eyes red, skin damp with sweat, the pulse becomes weak and irregular, and at last from the increasing narrowness of the windpipe, the horse actually dies for want of breath.

TREATMENT.—The treatment is by no means difficult or complicated. Give the SPECIFIC, A A, for INFLAMMATION, fifteen drops every hour during the violence of the disease, and until the difficult breathing has abated and the animal becomes comparatively easy. Then the intervals may be prolonged to two and then to three hours, or more until entire relief is obtained. If a cough remains the E E, may be given in alternation with the A A, to complete the cure.

Should the windpipe be very sore to the touch outside, it may be occasionally bathed with THE MARVEL with advantage.

Sore Throat or Quinzy.

This form of disease often occurs in connection with, or as a mere symptom of a *cold* or *Bronchitis*, and only requires to be treated in connection with those affections. But it sometimes appears as a more isolated disease, and deserves consideration accordingly, the affection involving the food pipe and the surrounding tissues more than the windpipe.

SYMPTOMS.—The throat is quite hot, painful, swelled on the outside; it is painful also internally, and the horse has difficulty in swallowing his food; he "quids" it, that is, partly chews and then drops it; refuses to drink, musses about in the water or swallows with evident reluctance and pain; the glands under the jaw and below the ears are swelled, hard, and painful, and sometimes maturate; sometimes in swallowing fluid it returns again by the nose; slaver drops from the mouth; as the swelling of the inside of the throat about the top of the windpipe increases, the breathing becomes more and more difficult, and the animal at times seems nearly suffocated; and there is always fever.

TREATMENT.—Commence with the SPECIFIC A A, for INFLAMMATIONS, of which give fifteen drops every two hours; after say three doses give the SPECIFIC C C, in alternation with the A A, at intervals of three hours, and so continue until the disease is conquered. Bathing the outside of the throat with THE MARVEL will be of essential advantage, and will expedite the cure.

Nasal Gleet.

This is the term applied to an old long-standing running from the nose. It arises from a morbid condition of the lining membrane of the nose, and is often the result of a badly treated or neglected cold, especially in old worn out horses, and is similar to catarrh in the human species. Sometimes a diseased tooth in the upper jaw may give rise to a similar discharge, but this is not a true gleet.

SYMPTOMS.—The discharge is yellowish or like cream and in some cases greenish. It may be discharged in clots, or of some thickness, constantly flowing, or snorted out in quantities; it may come from both nostrils, but generally only from the left. The glands under the left jaw are often fixed, hard, and painful. The membrane of the nose has a lead color. The discharge may stop for a time, and then come on again, more profuse than before. After continuing a long time, the animal becomes thin and poor, and may finally die of glanders.

TREATMENT.—The SPECIFIC for DISTEMPER, NASAL GLEET, C C, should be given, a dose of fifteen drops, three times per day. It will be found quite sufficient to entirely control and finally arrest it in recent cases, and will not fail to benefit even the most inveterate.

Pleurisy, Pneumonia, Pleuro-Pneumonia, Inflammation of the Chest.

The pleura is the delicate serous membrane, covering the lungs with one surface, and lining the cavity of the chest with the other. Systematic writers treat of the inflammation of this membrane, Pleurisy, and that of the substance of the lungs, Pneumonia, separately. But as this rarely occurs in fact, and leads to no practical result in the treatment, and indeed can be rarely detected before death, I prefer the more practical course of treating them together. An inflammation of the lungs rarely or never remains so, but eventually involves the pleura more or less, and so an inflammation of the pleura always involves more or less extensively, the pulmonary substance. The best name, and more common type of the disease, is hence PLEURO-PNEUMONIA.

CAUSES.—Catarrh Influenza, Cold, or bronchial irritation may either of them terminate in this disease if neglected, or from fresh exposure. A sudden transition from heat to cold; change from a warm stable to a colder one; neglect of the usual blanketing, or even of other comforts; hard and long riding against a cold wind in snowy weather; loitering in an exposed, bleak place, when the horse is fatigued and warm, without covering. It sometimes occurs when horses are suddenly turned out to grass, or when they have been taken up and turned into a very warm stable. Injuries, contusion, rupture, or great violence done to the chest, is quite sure to be followed by Pleürisy or Pleuro-Pneumonia.

SYMPTOMS.—For conveniences sake, we will indicate the symptoms of these two branches of the disease separately. Pleurisy invariably commences with shaking all over, followed by a hot, dry mouth, white coated tongue, red nose and eyes, low spirits, want of appetite, anxious look, and hard, quick, wiry pulse. The act of drawing the air *into the lungs* is short, and stops, or is cut off at a certain point, at which time the pain is felt; the act of forcing the air *from the lungs* is full and slow. The pain is increased by coughing and taking full breath which the horse will do if suddenly moved or frightened. If the inflamed side is pressed upon, he gives forth a sound like a grunt; the cough is short; the horse remains standing; the skin on the inflamed side is thrown into folds, and twitches are occasionally seen at the same place. The painfulness of the spaces between the ribs when pressed upon, is quite characteristic, and often exists to an intense degree. The horse shrinks from it with a low grunt, and tries to get away. The skin about the sides of the nostrils and at the ends of the mouth is wrinkled. The neck is lengthened, and nose thrust forward; the horse stands in a crouching manner, and seems uneasy, but does not move. As the disease advances, the pulse becomes more frequent, and afterwards smaller, until it can scarcely be felt; the breathing becomes quicker and more painful and catching, when the air is drawn into the lungs. Then by degrees, no catch is seen or grunt heard, the twitches are not observed, cold clammy sweats break out over the body, the horse appears dull and stupid, and death closes the scene.

The pleura, like all serous membranes, has a strong tendency to effusion, or exudation of fluid, during an inflammatory action and in the course of the disease this effusion, consisting of yellowish serum, is exuded, in quantities varying from a few ounces to a bucket-full. It occurs in all severe cases, and the fluid either is again absorbed, if in small quantity, or is the immediate cause of death, if in very large quantity, or a lesser amount may remain for a long time, impeding respiration, and forming an empyema or dropsy of the chest. When it exists, the breathing is always labored, and there is *œdema* or tumid swelling of some external part, generally the abdomen, chest, or point of the breast.

By listening with the ear against the chest, the progress of the effusion may be traced from below upward. Above it, will be heard the loud crackling respiration and grating peculiar to the disease; below, the dullness and stillness of the lung enveloped in fluid, the absence of sound, marks the line of the accumulated fluid its increase and diminution.

IN PNEUMONIA, the symptoms differ from Pleurisy, yet the difference manifests itself in this, that in *Pleurisy* there is more pain, and in *Pneumonia* more difficult breathing. Pneumonia is often a consequence of cold, bronchitis, or the termination of some disease of the air-passages, and may begin with symptoms of a cold—rough coat, want of appetite, low spirits, etc. In other cases, it begins with a shivering chill; the legs, ears, and skin are cold; the coat is rough; the nose pale and dry; quick pulse, which afterwards becomes frequent and full; breathing at first quick, then panting and heaving; the skin now becomes hot, except *the legs which remain very cold.* This is *a characteristic symptom and will never deceive;* the nose and eyes are red; mouth hot and dry; the eyes have a yellowish color, and the horse looks uneasy and restless.

As the disease extends, the breathing becomes more difficult, and is attended with heaving of the flanks; the nostrils are much widened; the nose and head held out; the neck lengthened; the fore-legs are fixed in one place, and spread apart; the nose and eyes have a dark blueish color; the face looks anxious and disturbed; *the legs* and ears are *very cold;* the legs seem fine, and the hair upon them glossy; the cough is more frequent, hard, and painful; the horse seems drowsy; there is no appetite; the dung is hard and covered with slime, and the urine high-colored and scanty.

In the last stage, the pulse is small, weak, and can scarcely be felt; the breathing is quicker and more difficult; the breath is very hot; the eyes and nose are lead-colored; the skin is cold, and clammy sweat breaks out upon it here and there; the mouth is cold; the tongue is coated; the teeth are ground every now and then, and twitches are occasionally seen. The eyes become more and more heavy, glassy, and dim; the strength becomes less and less; the horse leans against the stall or manger, or wanders around; he staggers and falls; tries to rise, but cannot; groans, struggles, and dies.

As an improvement takes place, the horse appears more natural, warmth returns to his extremities, his breathing is more free, pulse softer, fuller, and less frequent, cough easier, *and he lies down* quietly, and without uneasiness. These good symptons rarely or never deceive.

Placing the ear against the ribs, upon various parts of the chest, we may learn with some practice to distinguish the progress of inflammation. In the healthy lung, the air passes in with a slight, rustling murmer, quite characteristic, and which, once heard, will always be recognized. As the lung becomes inflamed, "crepitation" takes place, and we hear a sound, slightly cracking, like that made by salt thrown into the fire, or by rubbing the hair between the fingers close to the ear. As, by degrees, the lung becomes more intensely inflamed, it is more and more impervious to the air, until it becomes "hepatized" or solid, and gives no sound, and no resonance when percussed, or struck upon. These changes are interesting, and afford to the practiced ear clear indications of the state and progress of the disease.

PROGNOSIS.—Horses may get well in all stages of Pleuro-Pneumonia, except in very extensive hepatization, or solidification of the lung, when, if recovery occurs at all, it will be imperfect. The success has gained immensely under Homeopathic and Specific treatment, and hundreds of cases are thus saved, which would be lost under the best directed old school methods, to say nothing of the "hotch-potch" usually employed.

TREATMENT.—Give, the first twenty-four hours, the SPECIFIC for INFLAMMATION, A A, a dose of fifteen drops every two hours. After that, give the SPECIFIC for COUGH and INFLAMED LUNGS, E E, alternately with the A A, at intervals of two or three hours between the doses.

Continue this treatment steadily and uniformly by night, as well as by day, if the attack is severe, giving no other medicine, and making no deviation. After a day or two, with the remission of the more violent symptoms, the medicines for FEVER, A A, may be omitted entirely, and only the E E, given as also after the disease has turned, and during convalescence. After the horse has commenced to improve, a dose of the E E, every four hours during the day, will be sufficient to complete the cure. The treatment is the same whether symptoms of Pleurisy or Pneumonia predominate.

Stabling and food as under Bronchitis.

We should bear in mind that in all severe cases of this disease, resolution does not take place under four days, and if an improvement takes place in one, two, or three days, we should be satisfied. Rare indeed will be the cases that do not terminate favorably under the Specific Homeopathic practice, carefully applied.

CHAPTER V.

DISEASES OF THE DIGESTIVE ORGANS.

Dentition or Difficult Teething.

THE cutting or shedding of the teeth, and especially of the tushes, is sometimes attended with considerable disorder of the body. The animal either will not eat his food, or he has pain and difficulty in chewing it; the body grows thin; bowels are out of order; humors may break out in the skin. and there may be cough and slight fever present. The gum is hot, painful, and swelled.

TREATMENT.--Give the SPECIFIC for FEVER, A A, fifteen drops three times per day. This soon relieves the feverish irritation, and the tooth usually makes its way quiety to the surface. Nicking the gum directly over the tooth in the form of a cross is sometimes beneficial. If teeth are very slow in coming, showing an evident deficiency of bony deposit, an oyster-shell burned to lime, and broken or ground in his feed, will promote the growth and production of bone and be of service.

Diseased or Irregular Teeth.

Sometimes the teeth of a horse present irregularities. Some of the teeth are too long, or become ragged. As a consequence, the tongue or cheeks are wounded, and the horse eats imperfectly, has pain, drops or "quids" his food. Whenever this condition is found, if the difficulty does not mend itself, the long teeth should be extracted if loose, or be filed down, and the points of the ragged teeth smoothed off.

Decayed teeth produce similar symptoms. In addition, a bad smell exudes from the mouth; stringy saliva flows away in large quantities, and the eyes may be inflamed. If allowed to remain, the fang may become diseased, the socket and gum inflame, an abscess form, and a portion of the jaw-bone may die. If in the upper jaw, the matter may burst into the nose and be discharged. It is of bad smell and color, and has been mistaken for nasal gleet and glanders.

Examine carefully with the finger, and by feeling along the jaw, see if there is any swelling or indentation, or if there is any old stub or loosened tooth, a milk tooth that has been pushed one side, or down, or is loose, making the gum inflamed or painful and preventing the animal properly eating his food. If so remove the stub or loose tooth, or file off the ragged portion, so that the mouth may become sound and healthy. Sometimes a thick unhealthy discharge from the nostrils has been mistaken for glanders, when the real difficulty was from diseased teeth.

TREATMENT.—Draw out the diseased tooth, and give the SPECIFIC for INFLAMMATION, A A, each morning, and that for NASAL DISCHARGES, C C, at night; a dose of fifteen drops, for several days.

Lampas.

Occasionally the bars of the mouth swell and rise to a level with, and even beyond, the teeth, occasioning soreness, pain, and difficulty of eating. It is most common in young horses, in connection with the cutting and shedding of teeth, from congestion and the extension of the inflammation of the gums during this process It also occurs in old horses; for the growth of teeth in horses continues during life. Derangement of stomach, or worms, is sometimes connected with it.

TREATMENT.—The FEVER SPECIFIC, A A, may be required two or three times per day; a dose of fifteen drops This will soon relieve the irritation and swelling. Should there be any derangement of the digestive organs, a few doses of the SPECIFIC for INDIGESTION, J J, given morning and night, will promptly relieve not only the derangement of the stomach, but the Lampas also.

Swelling or soreness of the gums will be promptly cured by the use of the SPECIFIC J J, a dose of fifteen drops per day, or even morning and night.

The searing of the bars with a hot iron, as is sometimes practiced, by cruel and ignorant smiths can not be too strongly condemned. It tortures the horse to no purpose, renders the mouth callous, and destroys the delicacy and sensibility of a part upon which all the pleasure of driving and riding consists, while it is totally unnecessary.

Crib-Biting.

Much has been written upon crib-biting. It is generally regarded as a vicious habit but is, I think, connected more or less intimately with a mere morbid condition of the digestive organs. The horse stands with his neck bent, lays hold of the manger with his teeth, and violently sucks in wind, and then again with a grunt belches it out. It frequently occurs when eating, and the food and a large amount of saliva is either again thrown into the manger or upon the ground. The habit is very inveterate, and said also to be taken or imitated by one horse from another. Wind sucking is a variety of the same thing.

TREATMENT.—The Specific for INDIGESTION, J J, should be given daily fifteen drops, or morning and night. Omit for a few days, and then go on again. In many cases the disease or habit may be cured entirely—in all, benefited. In any case it is better to remove the manger or rack, or whatever the animal cribs upon, and to feed the horse from a bucket, and also give the hay upon the floor. You thus break up the habit and remove the occasional cause, though an inveterate "criber" often becomes a "weaver."

Loss of Appetite.

Loss of appetite or diminished appetite is but a mere symptom of some more general affection. It is a symptom of almost every disease, and especially of every morbid condition of the digestive organs. There are cases, however, in which this seems the most prominent symptom; and the animal appears well in every other respect save that he does not eat. The teeth should be examined and, if needful, corrected. We should see also if the throat is sore. In general, loss of appetite will be found connected with a morbid or unhealthy condition of the digestive organs, and will yield to a few doses of the SPECIFIC for INDIGESTION, J J, fifteen drops morning and night. This is also the appropriate Specific for defective appetite or the weakness which often remains after acute disease.

Indigestion.—Hide-bound.

In consequence of over-feeding, bad food, suddenly changing the kind of food, working the horse too soon after eating too much food, or bad and uneven teeth, which prevent the horse from chewing his food well, the following condition presents itself:

SYMPTOMS.—The skin has the condition known as hide-bound; the horse sweats easily; he is weak, and can not work so long or with so much spirit as in health, he is thin and does not fatten; his tongue is foul; mouth slimy; the dung is dry, mixed with undigested oats, or it is slimy or bad-smelling; the water, is varible, scanty and thick; or clear and abundant, and there is a short, frequent cough. Sometimes he eats very greedily, and at others will eat nothing placed before him, or will take one kind of food and leave another, or he likes dirty straw or his bedding better than the best oats or hay, or, in some instances, his morbid appetite leads him to lick the wall or eat plaster from it.

TREATMENT.—Correct the feeding Give not too much, and only that most acceptable at first. Give fifteen drops of the SPECIFIC for INDIGESTION, J J, morning and night. It will likewise correct the rough staring coat which accompanies this unthrifty condition.

Stomach-Staggers.

The cause of this condition is excessive repletion and distension of the stomach with undigested food. It occurs also from weakness of the stomach, bad condition; old age, eating too much dry food after long fasting, violent or hard work immediately after a full meal. These causes prevent the digestion and passage of the food, and, as a result, congestion of the brain and staggers.

SYMPTOMS.—Are similar to those of mad staggers at the commencement, and are principally known from each other by the manner in which the disease comes on. The horse is found dull and sleepy; perhaps still eating slowly and carelessly; or he is fast asleep, the head upon the manger, or against the wall, or between his legs; the breathing is slow and labored; the pulse slower than in health; the eyes closed or nearly so; slight convulsions occur; the nose and eyes look yellow; he will sometimes paw on the ground, look around to his flanks, or lie down and roll, showing that he is griped and uneasy. All these symptoms become worse by degrees until the animal dies.

TREATMENT.—Give the SPECIFIC for INDIGESTION, J J, fifteen drops every hour, and continue this treatment until relieved. But if the staggers increase or show more tendency to engorgement of the brain, the SPECIFIC for STAGGERS, A A, should be alternated with that first mentioned, in doses of fifteen drops, repeated every hour at first and then at longer intervals, and the two may be continued in this manner until relief is obtained. If the dung should be dry, scanty, or suppressed, large and frequent injections of tepid water will be of great value.

Colic.

This is one of the most common diseases of the horse. The passage of food along the bowels is effected by the alternate contraction and relaxation of the muscular coat of the intestines. Hence it is easy to perceive that flatulent or irritating food, food in too large quantities, large quantities of green food that produce much gas, masses of hard, dry dung, or sudden chill upon the warm skin, all may produce irregular contraction of the intestines, and hence produce pain and colic. Tumors, worms, and stones also produce the same result.

SYMPTOMS.—In colic the attack begins suddenly. The animal is uneasy; shifts his position, paws or stamps the ground, kicks his belly with his hind feet, looks frequently at his flanks, groans, falls upon the ground and rolls about violently, or lies on his back, in which posture he remains for a short time seeming quiet and free from pain. Soon however, the pain comes on again, even with symptoms of greater intensity than before. He throws himself widely about, careless of the injuries he receives during these moments of agony and tossing. He grinds his teeth, bites the manger, and looks towards his flanks with a wild, anxious expression. If he improves, the paroxysms become less frequent and less violent, and free intervals longer, until entire relief; or if worse, the pain becomes more and more intense, paroxysms more frequent until there is no free intervals; inflammation results, the ears and legs become cold, pulse small and wiry, and the animal dies from the results of the inflammation.

Many of the symptoms of colic are similar to those of inflammation of the bowels, and as the latter is by far the most formidable disease, we will endeavor to distinguish them, so as to avoid mistake.

The attack of colic is sudden, while that of inflammation is more gradual. In colic, the pulse is rarely quickened, and never so early in the disease, while in inflammation it is very quick and small even from the first.

In colic, the legs and ears are of the natural temperature. In inflammation, they are cold. In colic, there is relief from rubbing the bowels and from motion. In inflammation the bowels are very tender, and motion vastly augments the pain. In colic, there are intervals of rest, while in inflammation there is constant pain. In colic, the strength is scarcely affected, while in inflammation there is great and rapidly increasing weakness.

Attention to these peculiarities will enable one to distinguish between the two diseases, and to avoid error in the treatment.

TREATMENT.—We have in the SPECIFIC for COLIC, F F, a remedy which rarely fails to arrest this disease. Give fifteen drops on the tongue, and repeat the doses every half or even quarter of an hour until relieved, omitting the medicine altogether, or giving it at longer intervals as soon as the amendment is perceived.

If at the commencement or during the progress of the disease, fever and inflammatory symptoms should also exist, then alternate the FEVER SPECIFIC, A A, with that for colic, F F, at the intervals mentioned.

If the attack has clearly been occasioned by an *over feed* or by bad, heavy, indigestible food, it will be best to alternate the SPECIFIC for INDIGESTION, J J, with that for COLIC, F F, at the intervals directed.

The colic not unfrequently comes from the kidneys which may be suspected by the horse making frequent attempts at staling, or his passing scanty, thick or bloody urine. In these cases give the H H, SPECIFIC for kidney disease, fifteen drops every half-hour, alone or in alternation with the A A.

Should there be suspicion that Bots or Worms are an exciting cause, the WORM SPECIFIC D D, may be alternated with that for COLIC F F, fifteen drops every half-hour or hour.

N. B.—In cases of colic the greatest danger and the worst possible fault is injudicious haste and giving *too many and improper things.* Thousands of horses are killed by the drugs given to cure colic where one dies of the disease itself. Give only the Specific Remedies, and at the intervals as directed, however urgent as the case may appear. Your success and safety are in following the directions implicitly.

Tympanitis, Drum-Belly or Wind-Colic.

This is merely a form of colic characterized by an enormous production of flatulence. The pain is sharper, the animal more furious and violent than in ordinary colic; the belly on both sides is more or less swelled with wind; there are rumbling noises and frequent discharges of wind. It is usually the result of eating or gorging with green flatulent food.

TREATMENT.—Give fifteen drops of the SPECIFIC for COLIC F F, every half-hour, or even more frequently if the case is very urgent. It will soon be relieved. Afterwards a few doses of SPECIFIC J J, fifteen drops morning and night will be of benefit.

Enteritis, Inflammation of the Bowels, Red Colic.

There are two varieties of this disease, one in which the external coats of the intestines are inflamed, and attended with constipation, and the other, in which there is irritation of the internal mucus surface of the intestines, and attended with purging.

The most frequent CAUSE is sudden cold upon a warm, perspiring skin, or even a cold drink, when very hot; over-fed horses, subjected to long and severe exercise, are most liable to it ; stones and hard dung in the bowels ; and especially colic badly treated, and drugged with all sorts of medicines, often terminates in Inflammation of the Bowels.

SYMPTOMS.—The disease begins, in most cases, with dullness, heavy eyes ; staring coat ; restlessness and moving about from one place to another ; the pulse and breathing are both quickened ; no appetite. Some cases begin with colic others with shivering. The animal paws, kicks, and rolls about in the most violent manner at first ; often strains and tries to pass water, but either none or only a few drops come away ; the pain is most intense, and does not cease for an instant, and is increased by pressure and moving about ; the belly is hot, tucked up, and hard, unless there is wind in the bowels, when it will be more or less swelled ; the bowels are very costive, though small, hard, dry masses may be passed, except in cases where the internal surface, or mucus membrane is the seat of disease, in which case, small purging bloody stools are frequently passed ; the legs and ears are intensely cold ; the pulse small and hard ; and sweat in the latter stages breaks out all over. Still further on, the pulse becomes smaller and weaker, until it can scarcely be felt ; the breathing is quick, irregular, and attended with sighs ; the skin is covered with a cold clammy sweat ; the eyes seem to have lost their power of seeing, he becomes very weak, and trembles all over ; convulsions come on, and death soon follows.

Consider carefully the distinctions between Colic and Inflammation, as given under the article on Colic.

TREATMENT.—As early as possible, give the SPECIFIC for INFLAMMATION, A A, fifteen drops, and repeat the doses every half hour. After the animal is somewhat relieved, continue the medicine at longer intervals. If not better in two hours, the SPECIFIC for COLIC, F F, may be alternated with that for Inflammation, at the intervals mentioned. This will be especially indicated if there should be frequent purging small stools, blood-stained or otherwise After the inflammatory symptoms have subsided, a dose or two of the SPECIFIC J J, for INDIGESTION, will complete the cure.

N. B.—As constipation exists in inflammation of the bowels, many persons suppose it to be the cause of the disease, and resort to the most desperate means to remove it. This is all wrong. Remove the inflammation, and the bowels will then move of themselves, while the balls and cathartics administered during the inflammation will only increase the difficulty, and often even prevent the possibility of a cure.

Peritonitis, Inflammation of the Peritoneum.

The delicate membrane lining the abdominal cavity, and covering the parts within it, is termed the peritoneum, and is occasionally the subject of inflammation.

It not unfrequently follows the gelding of the horse, especially if he is too soon afterwards turned out to grass, or during cold and wet weather. Exposure to cold, standing in draughts of air, or drinking cold water, may produce it; and it follows a stab in the belly or a rupture of some of the viscera, and the flow of the contents into the abdomen.

SYMPTOMS.—A few days after cutting the colt, the yard and sheath will be found swelled and painful; little or no matter flows from the cut; the animal is restless and uneasy; the body is painful when pressed against, and is swelled with watery fluid; the legs are cold; the bowels are bound; the skin is rough and dry; no food is eaten; if loose, he rests his hind-quarters on the side of the stall; the swelling in the breast, legs, and sheath increases; the breathing becomes quick and painful; the pulse hard, quick, and by degrees small and weak. These gradually become worse, until the animal dies.

There is a slow form of this disease, as follows: poor appetite; low spirits; uneasiness; occasional pawing the ground; looking at the belly and groaning; belly painful when pressed upon, and tucked up; quick breathing; small weak pulse; bound bowels; awkward way of walking with the hind-legs; mouth dry and bad smelling; body thin; coat staring and unthrifty; urine scanty; weakness. As the disease advances, the abdomen fills with a watery fluid, and the disease terminates as dropsy.

TREATMENT.—From the commencement, the SPECIFIC for INFLAMMATION, A A, is the most important remedy, and may be given fifteen drops every two hours, during the more urgent symptoms, and then at longer intervals for the acute form.

If there should be purging, alternate the SPECIFIC for DYSENTERY, F F, with that for INFLAMMATION, A A, at intervals of two hours, and then less frequently as the disease improves.

In the slow form of the disease, the alternate use of the SPECIFIC for INDIGESTION, J J, and that for COLIC, F F, four times per day, will be found most effectual in preventing a termination in dropsy, and in restoring the animal.

Diarrhea, Purging, Scouring, Looseness.

Green food; new hay; worms; excess of bile; cold air or water; quick work, after much eating or drinking, may produce diarrhea. So does aloes, or other purges, which may even kill a horse.

SYMPTOMS.—Frequent and abundant discharge of slime, and dung mixed with slime; pain in the bowels, causing the horse to paw and stamp, look at his sides, and roll about violently; his face is anxious; cold sweat breaks out; his legs and ears are cold; the pulse becomes small and weak, the breathing becomes quickened; body wastes rapidly and alarmingly, and no food is taken. Death, at times occurs from sheer exhaustion.

TREATMENT.—Give the SPECIFIC for Diarrhea, F F, fifteen drops four times per day. It will generally promptly relieve. In some cases a dose of the SPECIFIC for Indigestion, J J, will be of value.

Dysentery, Flux.

Dysentery is most liable to occur in horses in good condition, and is caused by change of food, and over-work, or sudden exposure to cold and wet.

SYMPTOMS.—There are frequent passages of slimy, bad smelling, fatty matter, like "molten grease," which is more or less mixed or stained with blood. This is passed off with much straining and effort, and with frequent unsuccessful straining or attempts to effect a passage. The mouth is hot and dry, the legs cold, the breathing quick, no food is taken, the pulse is small and weak, there is great thirst, and the horse becomes thin and weak. Not unfrequently, in straining, the gut is thrust out of the fundament.

TREATMENT.—Should there be considerable heat and fever, it will be as well, or better, to give a few doses, fifteen drops of the SPECIFIC for FEVER A A, at intervals of two hours.

Then after two or three doses of A A, give the SPECIFIC for Dysentery, F F, a dose of fifteen drops, every two hours, until relieved. As the disease improves the intervals between the doses may be increased. The persevering use of the remedy will cure all cases.

Jaundice, Yellows, Diseased Liver.

Young horses rarely have diseased livers, but at the age of eight or nine years, the disease is more common, and, in some cases, quite suddenly, the covering of the liver gives way, and symptoms of fatal peritonitis appear.

SYMPTOMS.—Jaundice, or Yellows, is more frequent, and is marked thus: The animal is dull, sleepy, and unwilling to move; he eats little or nothing; the coat stares; the urine is scanty; the dung dark-colored and in lumps. The nose, tongue, eyes, and mouth becomes yellow, from the abundance of bile in the blood The dung becomes mixed with bile, and covered with slime; the urine is very thick, dark-colored, and full of bile. The right side is painful when pressed against, and the horse looks towards it; he may be lame in the right fore-leg, or paw the ground with it. These symptoms may increase, and cough, quick breathing, and full quick pulse, be added, which afterwards becomes quite weak and slow, and the legs very cold. He then becomes more and more dull, stupid, and sleepy, staggers, falls to the ground, and dies.

TREATMENT.—Rarely will anything more be required than the SPECIFIC for JAUNDICE, J J, of which a dose of fifteen drops may be given, four times per day.

Should there be heat fever, or inflammatory symptoms, a few doses of the FEVER SPECIFIC, A A, will be proper, not merely for the heat and fever, but for the obstruction of the liver as well. In severe cases, these two remedies may be alternated with the most brilliant success, even when there is no fever apparent. Give fifteen drops every four hours, alternately, first A A, next J J, and so on.

Costiveness, Bound Bowels.

This is usually a mere symptom of some other disease, upon the removal of which the costiveness disappears. But sometimes, in consequence of dry food deficient action of the liver, want of exercise, or a paralytic condition of the digestive organs, it may require attention.

TREATMENT.—The animal should have regular exercise, green food or bran-mashes night and morning, with, but little oats, or other heating or dry food. Give night and morning, fifteen drops of the SPECIFIC for INDIGESTION, J J, and the condition will soon be corrected.

Bots and Worms.

Bots, in the horse, like worms in the human system have usually a great many sins to answer for, which are really chargeable elsewhere. It is a principle in the economy of nature, that one animal should feed upon or live within another, and hence every animal and almost every organ also, has its peculiar parasite or inhabitant. Such parasites are rarely injurious In an unhealthy condition of the system, they may unduly accumulate, and occasion some inconvenience, but they rarely feed upon the surface to which they are attached, but only upon the contents of the organs in which they exist.

The history of the bot, the most formidable of horse parasites, is as follows. Towards the close of autumn, the female gad-fly, (octrus equi,) fixes its eggs upon the hair of the horse legs, by means of a sticky substance, exuded with the egg. By means of the horse's tongue and lips, these eggs are carried to the mouth, and so on down to the stomach, where the eggs, farther developed in the form of grubs, are attached, by means of their hooks, to the sides of the organ, while their heads remain floating in its fluids, upon which it feeds. Having arrived at maturity, they are separated, pass along the intestines, and are expelled with the dung, after which they again burst the shell, and rise in the summer in the form of the gad-fly.

SYMPTOMS.—Some horses are supposed to suffer much from bots, while others, in the most perfect health, have an abundance of them. Often there are no symptoms to indicate their presence, but generally, when in great numbers, the horse loses flesh and strength, until he becomes a skeleton, and can scarcely move about; he has turns of griping pains in the belly; eats and drinks greedily; the oats pass off undigested, and the dung has a bad smell. The only sure criterion of the existence of bots or worms is their presence, hanging about the anus, or mixed with the dung of the animal.

There are also the *long round worms*, similar to the common earth worm, and the *small pin worm*, half an inch or more in length, which often causes itching and uneasiness at the anus.

TREATMENT.—To eradicate worms or bots from the system, give fifteen drops of the WORM SPECIFIC, D D, each night and morning, with regular and healthy feed, and the worm symptoms will soon disappear.

For Colic or belly-ache, when supposed to be from bots, give fifteen drops of the SPECIFIC for BOTS, D D, alternately with that for FEVER, A A, every half-hour or hour, according to the urgency of the case. A few doses will usually relieve.

IN OBSTINATE CASES, when the Bots seem to be constitutional, give fifteen drops of the SPECIFIC, D D, every morning, and the same of J J, for Unthriftiness, every night, and so continue until good health is established.

CHAPTER VI.

DISEASES OF THE URINARY ORGAN.

Nephritis, Inflammation of the Kidneys.

THE Kidneys are not unfrequently the subject of inflammation in the horse. It may be induced by powerful or repeated diuretics, such as saltpeter, which is a most dangerous medicine, or from hard and long riding by a heavy rider, or heavy weights; or by leaping or being suddenly pulled up on his haunches, the inflammation being propagated from the lumbar muscles to the kidneys, or by exposure to cold and wet, by rain dripping upon his loins during exercise, and especially if these organs have been previously weakened.

SYMPTOMS.—The early symptoms are those of fever, the pulse full, hard, and quickened afterward becomes small and weak; the horse looks around anxiously at his flanks; stands with his hind-legs wide apart; is unwilling to lie down; straddles as he walks; expresses pain in turning; the back is somewhat arched; he shrinks when the loins are pressed upon, and there is some degree of heat felt there. The urine is voided in small quantities; frequently is high-colored, and sometimes bloody; and there is frequent and often violent effort and straining, but the discharge is very small, sometimes suppressed.

TREATMENT.—Give fifteen drops of the SPECIFIC for INFLAMED KIDNEYS, H H, and repeat every two hours.

Should there be very high fever, great heat, etc., the SPECIFIC for INFLAMMATION, A A, may be alternated with it, giving fifteen drops every intermediate hour in urgent cases, but in general the first-named SPECIFIC will be quite sufficient, and should be continued at prolonged intervals to entire recovery. But a few doses will be required to show us the great value and efficacy of the remedy.

Cistitis, Inflammation of the Bladder.

This disease is usually the result of giving diuretics, such as saltpeter, cantharides, or similar irritating medicines. It may also be the effect of a cold and exposure, or of a stone in the bladder, and the disease may occupy the neck of the bladder, or the organ itself. The symptoms are similar to that of Inflammation of the Kidneys; the horse makes frequent and painful attempts to stale, but passes only a few drops of water at a time. The bladder can not retain the urine from its excessive irritability, so that the attempt to void it is constantly going on. The urine may be clear, or mixed with mucus, or stained with blood.

The TREATMENT is the same as for Inflammation of the Kidneys, the SPECIFIC for that disease, H H, being given every two hours, in doses of fifteen drops, or less frequently, according to the urgency of the case. In some cases, the SPECIFIC for INFLAMMATION may be given in alternation, as for Inflammation of the Kidneys; but, in general, the remedy first mentioned, H H, will be found every way efficient and available.

Hematuria, or Bloody Urine.

This is usually a mere symptom of some other disease. Blows or a violent strain of the loins, some kinds of irritating plants, stones in the kidneys or bladder; ulceration of the bladder; Spanish flies given internally or administered as a blister,—may either of them produce bloody urine as a symptom.

The symptoms are: discharge of urine, mixed more or less with blood, or containing clots. When the blood is caused by some disease of the kidney, there is usually pain in walking, straddling of the hind-legs, and an awkward way of walking. If the blood comes from the kidneys, it will be intimately mixed with the urine; but if from the bladder, it will pass off with the last of the urine rather than the first.

TREATMENT.—Fifteen drops of the SPECIFIC for Urinary Diseases, H H, given three times per day, will generally promptly relieve. If dependent upon organic disease, more time may be required, but the remedy is the same. If it fails, give a large spoonful of THE MARVEL, poured upon the tongue three times per day.

Retention of Urine.

From holding the urine too long, cramp or spasm of the neck of the bladder, stone in the bladder, or other disease, which prevents the bladder contracting upon its contents, there may be retention, and the animal unable to void his urine.

The symptoms are similar to those in colic, but characterized, however, by the horse putting himself in the attitude of staling, and straining with great force, as in the act of passing water, without any, or very little, being discharged. This symptom may be present in cases of gripes or colic, the bladder acting in sympathy with the cramped intestine. All doubt may be removed by inserting the hand into the rectum, when the bladder, if full, will be found large, tense and full of water.

TREATMENT.—A few doses, fifteen drops each of the SPECIFIC for SUPPRESSED URINATION, H H, given at intervals of two hours, will not fail to relax the spasm and afford entire relief.

When it is the result of a stone in the bladder, the movements of the horse may for a time dislodge it, but an entire cure will only be effected by an operation, for which a veterinary surgeon must be consulted.

Scanty Urine.

This is a mere symptom of some other disease, such as fever, inflammation, or other morbid condition, or it may occur naturally, if there is diarrhea, loose bowels, or purging, and it always occurs in warm weather, when a horse is severely worked, from the large quantity of fluid exhaled from the skin and lungs.

A few doses, fifteen drops each of SPECIFIC for SCANTY URINATION, H H, will soon correct the condition, so far as the health of the animal requires. The SPECIFIC for INDIGESTION, J J, is likewise efficient.

Diuresis, Too Profuse Staling.

In consequence of bad food, such as kiln-dried oats, mow-burnt hay, or of such medicines as nitre or other diuretics, a horse may have an excessive flow of urine.

The symptoms are then as follows: the horse does not eat much, sweats easily, is soon tired, the bowels are costive, skin dry, aud coat rough, tongue white, and there is great thirst. The water is quite clear and milky, passed often, and in large quantities. As the disease advances, the horse eats nothing, he gets thinner and weaker every day; the dung is hard, lumpy and covered with slime; the hair stands on end, and the flow of urine becomes enormous. If not cured, death soon ensues.

TREATMENT.—The food must be changed, and none but the best given. Change of food is always of service under such circumstances.

Give fifteen drops of the SPECIFIC, J J, for INDIGESTION, four times per day. This will often be efficient; if it fails, you may try Phosphoric Acid, third attenuation, the same dose, three times per day.

Spinal Meningitis.

THIS disease is generally epidemic, induced by peculiar atmospheric conditions, and is favored by close, ill-ventilated stables. cold, chilly weather, overwork in mares during their periods of excitement, and more likely to appear among horses worked on Rail Roads or Omnibus lines, from the frequent stops and severe strain upon starting.

The earlier symptoms are dullness, indisposition to move, head hanging low, evident pain and stiffness on moving, and especially on turning tenderness and shrinking on pressure along some portion of, or along the entire spine, from the region of the kidneys forward.

The horse stands uneasily, and is easily pushed one side or over, or sways about. The back gives out, he falls down; no strength in the hind legs—cannot rise. The pulse at first is not increased, but becomes more rapid afterwards, and the urine is often scanty or suppressed, and dung dry, and the animal has from the first a distressed, suffering look.

The disease is frequently fatal in two or three days, but may continue much longer, and recoveries are usually quite slow.

TREATMENT.—Give the horse bran mashes, or carrot tea. and let him peck at hay. Let him have a wide stall, well littered or a loose box, reasonably warm, but with good air, and in cold weather well covered with blankets.

The A A, from the first is the principal remedy, and should be given every HALF HOUR a dose of

TEN TO FIFTEEN DROPS for the first six hours; then for twelve hours give it every hour, and afterward at intervals of two hours, and as the animal improves the intervals between doses may be prolonged to three or even four hours.

IF DURING THE DISEASE THE WATER should become VERY SCANTY, passed with difficulty or suppressed, then give the H H, in alternation with the A A, every two hours; that is, give A A, wait two hours and give H H; then wait two hours and again give A A, and so on, in doses of ten to fifteen drops until the secretion of water is established, when the H H, may be discontinued.

AFTER THE MORE URGENT STAGE HAS PASSED, and there yet remains WEAKNESS or PARALYSIS OF THE LOINS in any degree, the J J, is the remedy, and it may be given in the same doses, either in alternation with A A, if the acute symptoms have not entirely disappeared, or alone. For the remaining weakness, give at intervals of two to four hours at first, and afterwards four times per day. It is the special remedy for the paralysis and the convalescence.

The animal should not be exercised or worked too soon after recovery, for fear of relapse.

CHAPTER VII.

DISEASES OF THE FEET AND LEGS.

Laminitis, Inflammation of the Feet, or Founder.

This is one of the most frequent diseases of the horse, and one in which the resources of the Homeopathic art are very efficient. The sensible lamina or fleshy plates on the front and sides of the coffin-bone, are, like all other vascular structures, very liable to inflammation, particularly from violence or long continued action of the part. Hence, standing long in one position, as in voyages; battering or bruising the feet, in severe or long journeys; sudden changes from heat to cold, or from cold to heat, acting directly on the feet; standing in snow or cold water after a journey, are among the more common causes of this disease. It sometimes occurs as a mere transition of the disease from some other part, and occasionally from *excess of food or indigestible food*, or *food when heated*. Many cases of so-called FOUNDER, are really only attacks of *Acute Rheumatism;* hence consult what is said on that disease, and compare the two chapters for a better understanding of the subject.

SYMPTOMS —The disease generally begins with a shivering, shaking chill; the flanks heave; the breathing becomes quick and labored; the pulse full and frequent; the horse shifts his feet from one place to another, lies down and rises frequently, but does not paw the ground nor kick his belly; he will sometimes place his lips on the fevered feet, as if to tell where his pain is; he places his hind-legs under him, as if to take the weight of his body from the fore-feet; he moans or groans from the severity of the pain, and at last lies down, unable to stand upon the inflamed feet. The feet are intensely hot and painful. If one foot is taken up, he can scarcely stand upon the other and may tumble down. He does not like to get up from the ground, and is moved with difficulty from one place to another. If the disease be not arrested, matter may form inside the hoof, which is then thrown off.

The disease may exist in a more chronic form, coming on by degrees, and eventually resulting in the ruin of the horse.

It is more common to see it in a milder form than the first-mentioned, presenting the following symptoms: the horse is feverish, out of spirits, refuses to eat, cannot raise his limbs without evincing pain, trails his feet along with difficulty; cannot readily be made to go forward, or backward scarely at all. In the stable, horses bring the four feet near together, and there is no little difficulty in making them relinquish this attitude.

TREATMENT. " In the more severe cases, th shoes should be removed from the feet, and th hoof pared down until the horn yields to the pressur of the thumb. Give the horse rest, and allow hir to lie down, wrap the hoofs in cloths soaked in wa ter, and renew them from time to time.

If the die ease is from the feet having been battered by lon driving or riding, bathing them with the MARVEL c ARNICA will be of great value.

In some cases, cold poultice, made of mashed turnips or carrots, i of excellent service.

The remedy for all forms of this disease, is th SPECIFIC for FOUNDER, B B, of which a dose of fi teen drops may be given, every three hours, in acui cases, with the best possible effect. Should thei be quite high fever, the horse down, or scarcely abl to move, the SPECIFIC for FEVER, A A, may be a ternatecl wi h that for FOUNDER, B B, as often; every two hours, and after the force of the diseas has abated, the SPECIFIC B B, may be continue alone at increasing intervals, until entire restor tion.

When the disease is clearly traceable to over-fed ing, the SPECIFIC for FOUNDER, B B, and that f"

INDIGESTION, J J, may be alternated from the fin every three or four hours, in doses of fifteen drop In case of chronic Founder, the SPECIFIC f" FOUNDER, B B, should be given, a dose of fiftec drops each morning and night, and the treatme continued for some time. An occasional dose the SPECIFIC for INDIGESTION, J J, will be useful; a constitutional intercurrent remedy, and may 1 given at noon, while the SPECIFIC B B, is give morning and night.

Navicular Joint Disease.

This disease is far more frequent than is usually supposed, and many horses are ruined by it, the lameness being generally referred to the shoulder or tc some other part not at all in fault.

Behind and beneath the lower pastern-bone in the heel of the horse, and behind and above the heel of the coffin-bone, is a small bone called the navicular, or shuttlebone. It is so placed as to strengthen the union between the lower pastern and coffin-bone, and to enable the flexor tendon which passes over it, to be inserted into the bottom of the coffin bone, to act with more advantage. It thus forms a kind of joint with that tendon. There is a great deal of weight thrown on this bone and from this navicular bone on the tendon, and there is considerable motion or play between them in the bending and extension of the pasterns.

It is easy to conceive, that from sudden concussion or from rapid and over-strained motion, and at a time when, from rest and relaxation, the parts have not adapted themselves to the violent motion required, there may be excessive play between the bone and tendon, and the delicate membrane which covers the bone or the cartilage of the bone, may become bruised, inflamed and injured or destroyed, and that all the painful effects of an inflamed and open joint may result, and the horse be incurably lame. Numerous dissections have shown that this joint thus formed by the tendon and bone, has been the frequent and almost invariable seat of these obscure lamenesses. The membrane covering the cartilage becomes inflamed and ulcerated; the cartilage itself is ulcerated and eaten away, the bone has become carious, and bony adhesions have taken place between the navicular and pastern and coffin-bones, and this part of the foot has become completely disorganized and useless.

SYMPTOMS.—The degree of lameness is various; the horse may show lameness the first hundred steps, or the first mile or two, and then less or scarcely at all; he is inclined to "point" or keep the affected foot in advance of the other when standing; he may show lameness on stone or pavement and not on turf or ground; if both feet are badly affected, the horse favors his heels, has short action, and wears away the toes of his shoes, leaving the heels undiminished in thickness; the hind-feet may be kept well under him to diminish the pressure upon the fore-feet; in the stable, he is mostly lying down; heat of the foot and heel, especially the heel.

TREATMENT.—In the earlier stages when there exists only irritation and inflammation, and no changes of structure or disorganizations have yet occurred, the SPECIFIC for STRAINS or INJURIES, B B, together with cold fermentations kept to the foot, will be found sufficient. Give a dose of fifteen drops four times per day

In more extreme or advanced cases, the sole should be pared down and the quarters rasped, and shoe worn without nails on the inner quarter, to unbind as far as possible the imprisoned bone, and the foot kept in a bran poultice until the heat is allayed, then substitute this for the cold fermentation, keeping up the use of the SPECIFIC, B B, as above indicated. These will be successful in the incipient or milder stages of the disease.

Sand Crack, Quarter Crack.

This is a separation of the fibers of the hoof from above downward—rarely crosswise. The best treatment is to drill two holes through *each side of the crack* and then pass copper or iron wire through them. Both ends of the wire are then to be drawn and clinched down and fastened in the same way as the nails in shoeing. The crack itself is then to be filled with cobbler's wax after having been thoroughly cleaned out. Give also, morning and night, ten drops of the SPECIFIC, J J, to promote the growth of the hoof.

A yet better method is to properly prepare a *horse shoe nail* by cutting *bards along in it, from head to point.* Then drive the nail from one side of the crack through to and beyond the other at least half an inch from the crack. The clinching of the point of the nail will drive the bards back and firmly fasten them, and the head and point may be filed down and smoothed off. A long crack should have two nails. The shoe should be so fitted and the hoof so pared away, as to *take the bearing off from the cracked portion,* and as the hoof again grows down, it should be again *cut away between* the *hoof and shoe with a saw*, so as to keep the bearing of the cracked part of the hoof free. You thus rivet the broken parts together, and by taking off the strain allow the crack to grow out, and heal up. Of course a horse with a quarter crack should only be put to the most moderate work, if any, as violent exercise or hard work will be sure to aggravate and increase the difficulty, and may render a cure impossible.

Where a quarter crack occurs, some brittleness or defect of horny deposit or growth is presumably present, and to correct this and promote a healthy growth of the hoof, the SPECIFIC J J, should be given, a dose of fifteen drops morning and at night.

Corns.

A corn is a bruise upon the sole of the foot at the angle between the wall and the bar, and has this resemblance to the corn in the human subject, that it is produced by pressure and results in lameness. It may be caused by contracted feet; cutting away the bars; too thick-heeled shoes or weak flat feet; dirt getting between the shoe and heel of the foot; or from not having the foot sufficiently pared out.

SYMPTOMS—The pressure arising from these causes bursts the blood-vessels under the horn, so that the angle of the foot has a blood-red appearance, and feels softer than other portions of the horn; the place is painful, and, when pressed upon, the animal flinches, and there is more or less lameness. In some cases, matter will form, and unless a vent be made as early as possible, it will underrun the sole, or appear at the coronet and form a quittor.

TREATMENT.—The heel must be well pared out, and all dirt removed. Then apply Tincture of Arnica upon a bit of cotton, or THE MARVEL, if the Arniea is not at hand, tack on the shoe lightly, with the pressure off the sore heel, and a leather sole between it and the foot. But if matter has formed, remove the dead horn, make a good free vent, so the matter may freely discharge, foment the foot with hot water for an hour. Soak a bit of cotton in ARNICA or THE MARVEL, and apply it to the heel, and then place the foot in a large bran or turnip poultice. (See External Applications page 28.) Change the poultice and dressing each night and morning. In a few days the foot will be ready to shoe in the usual way using however a leather sole to keep out the dirt. Give also, each morning and night, a dose, ten drops, of the SPECIFIC for ULCERS, I I. If a quittor has formed, it should be treated as such.

Quittor.

This is a deep narrow ulcer opening upon the coronet, and leading into an abscess in the foot. It may be caused by treads, or overreaches, or corns, but most commonly from prick of a nail or other sharp substance. It is attended with more or less lameness; heat and pain in the foot, and discharge of matter from the open wound. But if it has been caused by the matter from a corn, the coronet above the heel will have upon it a hard painful swelling, which afterward becomes softer and larger.

TREATMENT.—If the quittor arises from a wound of the sole or prick, after the wounded part has been pared out and poulticed as directed in the article for prick in the foot, then with a probe gently find out the direction and number of pipes, and with a fine syringe, inject THE MARVEL of full strength, into the opening, two or three times per day. Change the poultice night and morning until no more matter flows, and the quittor begins to heal.

When it arises from a corn in the heel, and matter has got into the coronet, the swelling must be cut into and the discharge let out; then poultice night and morning, inject the MARVEL as before, rasp down the wall of the hoof until it yields to the pressure of the thumb, and put on a bar-shoe. Roll a bandage around the coronet to keep the dirt out from the quittor.

If there is some considerable heat and fever, the FEVER SPECIFIC, A A, may come in play, giving fifteen drops four times per day. But the SPECIFIC for ULCERS, I I, should be given, fifteen drops three times per day, at first, and then morning and night until the quittor is healed.

Prick in the Foot.

Sharp substances, such as nails, glass, pointed stones, or similar substances, not unfrequently penetrate the foot in traveling, or the shoe may be partly torn off, and the loosened nail be thrust into the foot, or a nail may go wrong in shoeing.

Heat, pain, lameness, and subsequent formation of matter, will be the result, unless the offending substance is removed in time and the injury cured.

TREATMENT.—With the hammer upon the nails, or by pressure with the pincers, ascertain where the horse feels pain, and the mischief lies. Take off the shoe, pare away the hoof around the injured part, until it yields to the thumb, follow the nail-hole to the bottom, and if newly done, a dark-colored dirty matter will flow out. Make a fair vent for the fluid, and if there is not much lameness, put a piece of cotton soaked in ARNICA OR THE MARVEL upon the pricked place, and tack the shoe lightly on with a sole leather and the usual stopping between it and the foot to prevent dirt getting into the wound.

If the injury has been of some days' standing and there is pain, heat, and lameness, matter has probably already formed, and may run under the sole or make its way to the coronet. In such cases make a good opening, remove all dead horn and that only; dress as before with ARNICA or THE MARVEL, and put the foot into a large bran or turnip poultice, which must be changed night and morning. Continue the poultices until the lameness is measurably subdued, and then dress with Arnica, and shoe as before.

During the treatment, give the SPECIFIC for INJURIES, B B, in doses of ten drops, every four, or six hours, according to the urgency of the case, and if there is much fever interpose a dose or two of the FEVER SPECIFIC, A A, as circumstances require.

Spavin.

This is an affection of the tendons, ligaments, and bursa connected with the hock. From a strain, violent exercise, or similar cause, an increased action is set up in these parts which glide upon each other, irritation results and the parts enlarge. Or, an exudation of serum occurs, tinged or not with blood, which may be absorbed afterward or remain for a long time a soft movable tumor; or by degrees an ossific or bony deposit takes place, resulting in a firm, hard, bony tumor. These several stages or degrees of the same common affection have been termed *Bog-Spavin*, *Blood-Spavin*, and *Bone-Spavin*. Wind-Galls and Thorough Pins are but local variations of the same essential condition—enlargements of the bursa and tendons of the joint. Spavin is essentially an inflammation of the ligamentous connections of the small metatarsal, with the internal cuneiform bone of the hock, yet the position of the swelling and ossific deposit may vary considerably. It usually shows itself on the inner and lower side of the hock at the lower portion of the joint. A careful comparison of the two legs with the eye and hand will best disclose the evil. "Sometimes it appears as a soft swelling of the femoral vein along the inner surface of the hock. Or again, as a hot. painful, laming swelling, extending from the posterior border of the hock downward, which may afterward become a hard bony tumor, insensible, causing the animal to limp only when making some exertion. Or, the swelling extends along the inner surface of the hock, oblong, a little broader above than below, bony, sometimes involving the entire joint, and occasioning more or less limping. Or, a soft round swelling over the whole internal surface of the hock, at first not impeding the horse's gait, but afterward becoming indurated and causing a rigidity of the hock and consequent lameness. Or, a hard osseous swelling at the upper and inner side of the femur, causing a lameness depending upon the extent to which the ligaments of the joints are involved. Or the muscles of the hind-quarters are not visibly affected, the horse does not limp, but simply raises one or both the hind limbs (for one is seldom affected alone) unnaturally high, with a spring, and puts them down again with a spasmodic twitching movement." (Spring-halt.)

At first the animal seems afraid to use one or the other of the hind-legs, and a little lameness is noticed on first starting off. Afterward when returning to the stable after exertion, the horse stands on the toe of the affected limb, and limps considerably on turning around and first commencing to walk; after moving a little, the lameness disappears, and only returns again after he has been standing some time. This will soon be followed by swelling.

CAUSES.—There is a predisposition to this affection in some families of horses, and when this predisposition exists, strains, violent exertion, over-work, a blow or other injury, readily develops the spavin.

Horses with high legs, from three to seven years of age, are most liable to it.

TREATMENT.—In the earlier stages, while the lameness is yet recent, and little or no swelling has appeared, bathing the joint with THE MARVEL or ARNICA, and giving the SPAVIN SPECIFIC, B B, night and morning, doses of fifteen drops will be sufficient to remove the lameness and generally prevent the swelling. When the swelling is still soft and recent, bathing the joint with THE MARVEL or ARNICA, and giving the SPAVIN SPECIFIC, B B, night and morning, will reduce the swelling and relieve the lameness.

In all other cases of spavin, whatever may be its particular form or situation, give fifteen drops of the SPECIFIC for SPAVIN, B B, each morning and night, see that the legs are well rubbed, with but moderate daily work or exercise. The pain, lameness, and subsequent exudation of bony matter depend upon the affection of the ligaments of the joint. This being relieved, the whole affection disappears. All recent and soft spavins may be successfully treated thus, and even the most inveterate ones will be relieved and benefited. It is not pretended or presumed that old chronic years' standing spavins, when there are extensive ossific dispositions or necrosis, are to be cured or caused to disappear by this or any medicine. But all those incipient cases may be thus cured.

Splint.

In consequence of an injury a bony tumor arises in the inside of the fore-leg below the knee; sometimes, though rarely, it is seen on the outside and even on the hind-legs. After having existed sometime they seldom occasion lameness except so situated as to interfere with the action of the tendons or ligaments of the legs. During the forming stage, the horse is lame because the periosteum or covering of the bone is inflamed, but after this has subsided and the bony exudation is thrown out, it disappears, except in the case above mentioned. In some cases in the beginning, the feet are hot and painful, the animal likes to remain lying down; and if only the fore-feet are affected, he puts them down with great care and evident pain, and there is general fever and suffering, which passes off with the more decided local manifestation. If the tumor is of some standing, it may be quite difficult or impossible to cause its disappearance. But happily these old hardened tumors seldom interfere with the essential usefulness of the animal.

TREATMENT.—In most cases if there is heat and feverish excitement of the system, give fifteen drops of the SPECIFIC for FEVER, A A, and that for SPAVIN, B B, alternately five times per day, that is, a dose of B B, morning, noon and night, and a dose of A A, at say 10 o'clock in the forenoon and at 3 in the afternoon until the heat and lameness are partially subdued, and then give the SPAVIN SPECIFIC, B B, morning and night, until the lameness and irritation have entirely subsided. Old cases will be benefited by a dose every day.

Ring Bone

Consists of an enlargement and ossific deposit (near the fetlock joint) in consequence of a strain and inflammatory action. It may appear on one or both sides of a foot, or completely surround it, giving rise to the name. One or more feet may be affected by it. It is generally recognized by a mere bony enlargement on one or both sides of the pastern, and the lameness is not very considerable. Sometimes not only the ligamentous but bony structures of the joint are involved, compromising the entire joint. A false step or strain of the articular ligaments are the usual immediate causes, to which a hereditary predisposition must be added.

At the commencement bathe the part with THE MARVEL or Arnica from day to day, and give fifteen drops of the SPECIFIC B B, for SPAVIN, three times per day. In chronic cases give a dose morning and night, or even only once per day. Cases of considerable standing will materially improve, and recent or fresh cases may be permanently restored.

Over-reach and Tread.

An over-reach is a bruise upon the heel of the fore-foot caused from the toe of the hind shoe. A tread is a bruise upon the inside coronet of a hind foot, caused by the shoe on the other foot treading upon it. It may also be caused by a fore shoe treading upon a hind coronet, as when the horse is backing. In either case quittor may form, or the death of the crushed coronet will leave the hoof altered in shape.

TREATMENT.—Remove the crushed and torn skin and horn; clip away the hair around the bruised part; wash it with water to remove the dirt; and foment it with hot water three times per day; after each fomentation wash it with THE MARVEL, and apply to it a piece of cotton soaked in the same. If matter is likely to form, put the foot in a large bran or turnip poultice, (See Introductory Section,) which is to be changed night and morning. Continue this until the pain and lameness become less, then dress it with THE MARVEL twice per day, and protect it from dirt by rolling a bandage over the dressing and round the top of the hoof. If quittor remains, it must be treated as directed for that disease. Give also, morning and night a dose of fifteen drops of the SPECIFIC for ULCERS, I I. Should there be much fever and pain, a dose or two of the FEVER SPECIFIC, A A, will be in place.

Thrush and Canker.

This disease is an inflammation of the lower surface of the sensible frog, which secretes matter of a peculiar offensive smell instead of healthy horn. The matter issues from the cleft of the frog. In a sound frog the cleft is shallow, but when contracted or otherwise diseased, the cleft deepens even to the sensible horn within, and through this the matter issues. Afterwards the discharge becomes more abundant and offensive; the frog wears off and a fresh growth of horn fails to appear. It then becomes thin, shriveled, contracted, and fissured; and as the disease extends, the matter becomes still more fetid, and may terminate in a yet more unmanageable form of disease, namely, *canker*. In Thrush the frog is painful when pressed upon by the thumb or pincers, or when the animal treads upon a stone. As a consequence of neglected thrush, the horn may separate from the sensible part of the foot, and unhealthy vegetations, proud-flesh, fungous matter, spring up, occupying a portion or the whole of the sole and frog, and finally involving frog, sole, and bars, in a mass of putrefaction, constituting the worst form of *canker*.

TREATMENT.—As thrush is often caused by uncleanliness and constant moisture of the feet, the greatest care must be taken to keep them dry and clean, and especially from dung and urine. If connected with contracted fore-feet, particular care must be given to shoeing.

The frog should be carefully pared down and all loose, ragged portions removed in order to prevent the accumulation of matter and dirt. The discharge wiped off by means of tow pressed down into the cleft with a thin piece of wood. Then smear the frog and cleft with a mixture composed of half an ounce of *sulphate of copper*, (blue vitriol), and six ounces of tar made into a paste. A small piece of tow dipped in this mixture should also be placed in the cleft, or in whatever part of the frog a sinus, hole or cleft exists. In bad cases repeat the dressing daily; in others, once in two or three days is sufficient. If the dressing is properly applied it will not fall out or admit the entrance of dirt. Should the frog be extensively diseased a bar-shoe may be necessary, and the dressing will then be kept in place by the cross-bar of iron, or a leather sole may be used under the shoe.

Throughout the treatment give fifteen drops of the SPECIFIC for ULCERS, I I, each morning, and fifteen drops of SPECIFIC, J J, for the growth of healthy hoof, every night.

CHAPTER VIII.

GENERAL DISEASES.

Rheumatism.

THIS is a far more common disease of the horse than has generally been supposed. It is quite common in old horses, and in younger ones that have been exposed or over-worked. Cold and damp, and exposure to draughts of cold air when heated, or during and after severe effort or work are among the most common causes.

SYMPTOMS.—It usually begins with a shivering chill, hot skin and mouth. The horse becomes lame and stiff all over, and several joints seem affected at once, so that he cannot move from the first, or else it soon becomes confined to one joint or leg; the joint or limb becomes very hot, swelled, and exceedingly painful; the pulse is quicker at one time than another, or stops now and then for a moment or two; the breathing is quick; sweats break out, and the animal becomes weak. When the disease attacks the fore-legs, farriers call it "chest-founder;" and when it attacks the loins, the back is raised and belly tucked up, and it is known as "loin-bound."

Rheumatism not unfrequently shifts from one place to another, especially if the animal is exposed to wet and cold.

TREATMENT.—If there should be considerable heat and fever, as is most commonly the case, give first the FEVER SPECIFIC, A A, a dose of fifteen drops every two or three hours, until the heat has been partially subdued, or until six doses have been given. Then alternate the SPECIFIC for RHEUMATISM, B B, with that for FEVER, A A, every three or four hours, a dose of fifteen drops until the animal is restored. If a limb or joint is painful, hot, and swelled, bathe it in THE MARVEL night and morning, and a flannel bandage applied to the limb will also be of great service, in addition to the internal medicines.

If at any time a horse shows symptoms of stiffness or lameness, fifteen drops of the RHEUMATIC SPECIFIC, B B, night and morning, will soon remove it.

Fever.

We understand by pure or idiopathic fever an increased arterial excitement, or increased frequency or force of the pulse, attended with heat, but without local inflammation. Symptomatic fever has the same heat and increased circulation attended with local inflammation or disorganization of some part, of which the fever is merely symptomatic. Bad management in the stable, impure and unwholesome food, bad air or confinement, are the usual causes of fevers.

SYMPTOMS.—IDIOPATHIC OR SIMPLE FEVER generally begins with a cold, shivering chill, or repeated chills, although this is not essential, or may readily be overlooked. The horse is dull, unwilling to move has a staring coat, and cold feet and legs. This is succeeded by warmth of the body; unequal distribution of warmth in the legs; one hot and the other three cold, or one unnaturally warm and the others unusually cold, but not the corpse like coldness of inflammation of the lungs; the pulse is soft, quick, and often indistinct; the breathing somewhat laborious; but no cough or pawing or looking at the flanks. The animal will scarcely eat, and is very costive. While the state of pure fever continues, the shivering fit returns every day at nearly the same hour, and that is succeeded by a warm one, and that often by a degree of perspiration; and these may alternate for several days until local inflammation appears or the fever subsides.

No horse dies of pure fever. If inflammation of the lungs, bowels, or feet does not set in, he will recover.

Symptomatic Fever is the result of some local inflammation or disorganization, or the result of injury, wound, etc. No organ or part can long seriously suffer without bringing the system into sympathetic suffering, which generally manifests itself by irritative fever, which of course disappears when the local irritation is removed.

TREATMENT.—In all cases of Fever, the FEVER SPECIFIC, A A, is the first and generally the only medicine required. Give a dose of fifteen drops at intervals of two or three hours at first, and by degrees at longer intervals, and not only will the fever be removed, but likewise all danger of its locating itself upon some organ or part of the system. Should such localization threaten, the FEVER SPECIFIC, A A, will still be the appropriate and best medicine. This SPECIFIC, A A, may be continued from day to day at intervals of three hours. Only if the fever assumes a *typhoid character*, with symptoms of great prostration or debility, give the SPECIFIC I I in alternation with the SPECIFIC A A, at the same intervals.

Distemper, or Strangles.

This is a disease incident to young horses, generally appearing between the third and fifth year, when the teeth are being shed, and is much more liable to appear in the Spring than at any other season of the year. Almost every horse has it, and but once in a lifetime. It is an idiopathic fever, followed by discharges in various parts of the body, generally under the jaw.

SYMPTOMS.—The disease begins with symptoms of a common cold; the horse is dull and depressed, eats little or no food, coughs now and then; the coat stares, the pulse is slightly quickened, the mouth becomes hot and dry, and afterward frothy fluid comes from it; the throat sore, the nose red, and matter flows from it. The glands under the jaw become swelled, hot, and painful, to such an extent as to cause "quidding," or dropping of food when eating, and there is so much difficulty of breathing, that the horse at times seems almost suffocated. The swelling, which occupies the center of the jaw, nearly filling its hollow, is a smooth uniform body (in distinction from glanders, which is uneven or knobby), becomes larger and softer until it bursts and matter flows out. From this time the animal begins to recover and soon gets well. In some cases, however, the horse does not get well so quickly, for after the abscess in the gland has burst others form upon the back, shoulders, legs, breast, or about the neck and jaws, and even internally. This form is termed irregular strangles. Strangles is said not to be contagious.

TREATMENT.—At the first when there is fever, hot and dry mouth, and glands swelled and painful, a few doses of the FEVER SPECIFIC, A A, given in doses of fifteen drops at intervals of four hours, or four times during the day, will reduce the fever and swelling, and the disease will run a milder course.

Afterward, the SPECIFIC for DISTEMPER, C C, should be given, a dose of fifteen drops three or four times per day during the height of the disease, and afterward at longer intervals, until entire restoration.

When the tumor under the jaw becomes hard, large, and painful, and suppuration is inevitable, a bran poultice applied warm, night and morning, will hasten suppuration so that it will break of itself or may be readily opened. The poultice may be secured to the place by an eight-tailed bandage tied in front over the nose and back of the ears, so as to keep the poultice in place.

Glanders and Farcy.

I prefer treating these two diseases in connection, persuaded they are one and the same—excited from a common cause, running a similar course; while the contagion of the one will produce the other, and *vice versa*. The disease is termed Glanders when it is principally confined to the head and nose, and called Farcy when manifesting itself in the lymphatics.

It is usually considered as the result of contagion, but want of food, bad food, bad keeping, impure air in too close stabling will generate it.

SYMPTOMS OF GLANDERS.—*Constant* discharge from one or both nostrils, more frequently from one, and that the left; the discharge is at first thin and watery, afterward thick like the white of egg. It may continue in this way for some time, or it soon becomes more mattery, sticky, then greenish or yellowish, or mixed with streaks of blood, and having a bad smell. Soon after this discharge is noticed, the glands under the jaw become painful and swollen, and one of them appears fixed to the jawbone. Then the membrane lining the inside of the nose has a yellowish or leaden color, which is considered characteristic of the disease; small bladders are noticed upon it, which afterward are changed to ulcers; these have sharp borders, and spread and deepen until the gristle and bones beneath become ulcerated. When ulcers appear upon the membrane of the nose, the constitution of the horse is evidently involved; he loses flesh; his belly is tucked up; coat unthrifty and the hair readily comes off; the appetite impaired; the strength fails; cough more or less urgent may be heard; the lungs become filled with abscesses, wasting goes on, and the animal soon dies.

FARCY.—Upon the face, lips, and other portions of the body, but especially upon the legs, hard, painful, and hot lumps are felt, which are called *Farcy buds*; they increase in size, with pain and heat, until the ulceration works through the skin and a thin discharge flows out. Between these lumps along the course of the lymphatics, hardened cords are felt; the groin, inside the thighs, and space between the forelegs and chest, become, from the tumefaction of these lymphatics, swelled and very painful; the legs are swelled, together with the usual discharge of glanders.

TREATMENT.—The SPECIFIC for DISTEMPER, C C, is the best remedy for either form of this disease, and should be given a dose of fifteen drops four times per day. During convalescence it need not be repeated so often.

Should a suspicious discharge appear at the nose, the C C given in doses of fifteen drops three times per day, will usually arrest it in a few days, and prevent further mischief.

A development of *Farcy* requires the same treatment as for *Glanders*. Give the SPECIFIC for DIS-

TEMPER, C C, four times per day. The horse should have good air and good wholesome food.

In some cases, the alternation of the SPECIFIC for ULCERS, I I, and that for DISTEMPER, C C, is very efficient, especially in cases of some standing.

N. B.—It should be remembered that a well-marked case of glanders is *highly contagious*. Not only may the disease be communicated to other animals, but the glandered matter coming in contact with a cut, abraded or sore surface in the human subject, will be liable to result as a very severe if not fatal case of poisoning. Prudence demands that we should handle such animals with great caution, and a thoroughly glandered animal had much better be killed at once than endanger other animals or the lives of human beings, and the more so as the chance of recovery in such a case is very remote.

Inflammation of the Lymphatics, or Weed.

In some rare cases horses suffer from inflammation of the lymphatics manifested by cord-like swellings along the course of these vessels. It may be brought on by sudden changes of food, cold and wet weather, sudden over-work after several days of rest, disordered stomach, standing in cold water, exposure to drafts of air, etc.

The SYMPTOMS are as follows: The attack is usually sudden, beginning with a cold shivering chill, followed by full, strong, and quick pulse, accelerated breathing; hot, dry mouth and general fever. The local manifestation is on one of the hind-legs, generally the left, or in rare instances, a fore leg may be affected. The leg is lifted from the ground, is hot and painful to the touch, and swells *from above downward.* The swelling increases rapidly, the leg becomes much larger than the other, the pain increases, and the leg is very sensitive to the touch. Several hard, round, and very painful cord-like swellings may be felt on the inside of the leg; these end in small hardish lumps, and are more painful than the cords. A watery fluid exudes from the skin, and may be seen in drops standing upon the hair.

TREATMENT.—At the commencement foment the limb for an hour, night and morning, with hot water, and afterward apply THE MARVEL freely. The horse should have plenty of exercise, and in most cases may be ordered to his work, continuing the medicine as hereinafter directed. Give three times per day fifteen drops of the FEVER SPECIFIC, A A. After a few days, the SPECIFIC for INDIGESTION, J J, may be alternated with the former with advantage. But in general the FEVER SPECIFIC, A A, will be entirely sufficient.

Purpura Hemorrhagica.

Some rare cases of this disease have been observed in the horse. It consists essentially of a decomposition of the blood, and loss of power in the capillary vessels, as the result of which, echymosed or black and blue spots appear on the surface, and upon the mucous membrane wherever it can be seen, hemorrhages occur from various parts of the body and are thrown off with the natural excretions. The inside of the nose is covered with purple spots, as also the inside of the lips. These spots vary in size, and are filled with dark-colored fluid blood, which exudes if they are punctured or scratched. There is diffused swelling over the system, showing itself at the eyelids, breast, flank, belly, quarters, and between the thighs, extending upward. It is attended with weakness and general prostration of the system, swelling and stiffening of the joints, and sloughing off of the membrane of the nose, or other parts.

TREATMENT.—The SPECIFIC for FEVER and INFLAMMATION, A A, will be found appropriate in all cases of this disease. Give a dose of fifteen drops three times per day. If there are hemorrhages from any organ, give half a gill of THE MARVEL three times per day, between doses of the SPECIFIC A A.

Give common food of good quality, less oats and hay but especially carrots and potatoes. The last are very serviceable in this disease.

PART II.

DISEASES OF CATTLE.

CHAPTER I.

GENERAL DISEASES.

Fever, Quarter Evil, Joint Murrain.

THIS disease, which is quite common, is known in different localities by various terms, as, *black quarter*, *quarter evil*, *joint murrain*, etc.

SYMPTOMS.—There are few premonitory symptoms. Often without any, or with slight indications of previous illness, the animal is found ill; the neck extended; the head brought as far as she can effect it into a horizontal position; the eyes protruded and red; the muzzle dry; the nostrils expanded; the breath hot; the root of the horns considerably so; the mouth partly open; the tongue enlarged, or apparently so; the pulse full, hard, and from 65 to 70; the breathing quickened and laborious; the flanks heaving violently, and the animal moaning in a low peculiar way.

Sometimes the animal is in full possession of her senses, but generally there is a degree of unconsciousness; she will stand for an hour or more without the slighest change of posture; can scarcely be induced to move, or when compelled to do so, staggers, and the staggering is principally referable to the hind-quarters; rumination has ceased, and the appetite is quite gone. After a time, the animal becomes more uneasy, yet it is oftener a change of position to ease the limb than a pawing; at length the animal lies down, or rather drops, gets up almost immediately, is soon down again, and debility rapidly increasing, she continues prostrate, sometimes comatose, and at others making fruitless attempts to rise. The symptoms rapidly increase, there is no intermission, and the animal dies in from twelve to twenty-four hours.

In the majority of cases, the animal seems to rally a little, and symptoms appear which give the local names of the disease. The beast attempts to get up; after some efforts it may succeed, but is sadly lame in one or both the hind-quarters. If not yet fallen, she is suddenly lame, so lame as scarcely to move, hence she has "joint *murrain*" or "*quarter evil.*"

Tenderness of the loins and back is one of the earliest symptoms and most to be dreaded. The animal will not bear even the slightest pressure on these parts. The case is worse if to this is added swellings about the shoulders, back, and loins, with a peculiar crackling noise, as if from deficient synovia or joint-oil. Worse than even this is the sudden appearance of hard scurfy patches of what seems to be dead skin. It is a dry gangrene, and the commencement of a process of sloughing extensive and rapid, to an almost inconceivable degree. This forms the "*black quarter*," with all its fearful characteristics.

Ulcers first appear about the belly, the quarters, and teats, but spread everywhere, and particularly about the muzzle and mouth. The tongue is blistered and ulcerated, and there is a discharge of sanious, offensive, or bloody fluid from the nose or mouth, or from both. The urine, previously high-colored, now becomes darker and bloody; the dung is streaked with blood, and all the excretions are excessively fetid. In this state the animal may remain some days, until it dies, a "mass of putridity."

TREATMENT.—Give fifteen or twenty drops of the SPECIFIC A A, for FEVER, every two hours, for the first twelve hours. This is more especially indicated for the fever, lameness, congestion, etc.

After the first twelve hours, unless there is decided improvement, give alternately the SPECIFIC I I for ULCERS, ROT, etc., in doses of twenty drops alternately with that for FEVER, every two or three hours, according to the urgency of the case. Continue this treatment without intermission or variation, prolonging the intervals between the doses as the animal improves.

Vesicular Epizootic.

This is an epidemic disease, which has at times invaded various sections of the country under somewhat varying forms, sometimes a lingering, and at others a rapidly fatal disease.

The symptoms are as follows. The premonitory indications are: dullness; impaired appetite; staring and harsh coat; the muzzle, ears, horns, etc., are cold at one time and hot at another; the beast shakes all over and feels uneasy, and does not associate with the other cows; the cud is not chewed as in health. Then the milk is found to be lessened, yellowish and thick; the bag is swollen, hot, and painful when touched; the back is arched, and she seems uneasy on her feet, and unwilling to move. This attracts attention to the feet, and they are found hot and painful; the hoof at the top is swelled, and a discharge runs from the heels; the eyes look dim, and tears run from them; the inside of the nose and whites of the eyes look red; the mouth is dry, and the membrane covering has little red spots in it, which rise into blisters upon it, over the whole mouth; they contain a fluid, and increase in size, finally burst, and a sore is left behind, which becomes a deep rugged ulcer. These blisters are also found upon the bag and about the hoofs, especially of the hind-legs; the hoofs may even fall off, the bones become diseased, and other grave results ensue. The appetite becomes more and more impaired; there is great weakness, wasting, discharge of stringy, bloody fluid from the mouth; offensive matter running from the nostrils; swollen face; bad breath; quick, grunting breathing; small, weak, quick pulse; dropsy of the belly and legs; purging, and death.

The causes, like those of all epidemic diseases, are involved in some mystery, yet it is indisputable that the disease, having occurred in a place or neighborhood, other cattle in the vicinity are more liable to be attacked, and those most so which are in contact or on the same place, and especially those that are poorly kept and housed, or at times exposed to bad weather, bad food, or other depressing influences. This rule applies to all epidemic diseases, whatever may be their particular form or manifestation.

TREATMENT.—To prevent the disease, if prevailing in the place or in the neighborhood, give fifteen drops of the SPECIFIC for DISTEMPER, C C, every night. This will tend to protect the system, or at least modify and diminish the force of an attack, should it come on.

To cure the disease: Give fifteen drops of the SPECIFIC for DISTEMPER, C C, every three hours, during the earlier stages of the disease, continuing so long as there is an improvement.

Should ulcerations have occurred, or blisters have formed on the mouth, bag, legs, etc, it will be better to alternate the SPECIFIC for ULCERS, I I, with that for DISTEMPER, C C, at intervals of three or four hours, during the height of the disease, and at longer intervals as the improvement progresses. The persevering use of the these SPECIFICS will save most cases.

Rheumatism.

This disease is almost invariably the consequence of cold and wet, or chill after over-exertion. The symptoms are as follows:

Dullness; loss of spirits; disinclination to move, and painful stiffness of the back or joints when moving; loss of appetite; pain in the back, manifested by the animal flinching when pressed upon; the joints, one or more, become affected, and the animal perfers to lie down, and cannot move without great pain and difficulty; the joints, or one or more of them, become swelled, and are also exceedingly hot and tender to the touch. In some cases, there is considerable heat and fever, in others it is but slight. The complaint is quite liable to return from exposure, changes of weather, or even the wind blowing from a different quarter. The disease not unfrequently changes from one joint or limb to another.

TREATMENT.—The SPECIFIC for RHEUMATISM B B, will cure all the usual forms of this disease, giving twenty drops three or four times per day, in severe cases, and morning and night in the mild ones.

When the disease is ushered in or attended with considerable heat and fever, either during its continuance, or from the first, the SPECIFIC for FEVER,

A A, in doses of twenty drops, should be alternated with that for RHEUMATISM, B B, at the intervals mentioned above. The use of these two remedies will control every form of this disease.

Lumbago.

This is merely a form of Rheumatism, locating itself upon the muscles of the loins. It may be mistaken for some other or different disease, and hence its symptoms should be known.

SYMPTOMS.—After some exposure, especially to cold or wet, or a draft of air, the cow will suddenly become lame of one leg, without other signs to explain the nature of the attack. Another leg may then be affected, while the first one seems better or quite well. Some pain and heat may be discovered in one of the joints; and then the muscles of the back show more clearly the location of the disease; or from the first the disease may be referable to this point; the animal yields and flinches when they are pressed upon, in consequence of the pain; the beast is not able to walk, or does so very stiffly and awkwardly, in consequence of increased pain from movement. These attacks may continue for a time, disappear and return again, in consequence of new exposure.

TREATMENT.—The SPECIFIC for RHEUMATISM, B B, should be given, a dose of twenty drops, three times per day. A few doses will promptly relieve.

Ophthalmia, Inflammation of the Eye.

Diseased and inflamed eyes in cattle may sometimes occur as a result of congestion, or from inflammation or a cold, but in general from an injury, the result of a blow of a whip, or stick, or from dirt or hay-seed, or some similar substance irritating the eye.

SYMPTOMS.—The eyelids are swelled and closed; tears flow in abundance; the eye shrinks from the light when the lids are opened; the white of the eye or conjunctiva is reddish or covered with red veins; the haw is also red and swollen; the eye itself is clouded and covered with a film.

TREATMENT.—Examine the eye for dirt, hay-seed, or other substances, and when found remove them. Bathe the eye with THE MARVEL diluted half and half with soft water, morning and night, until the more violent symptoms are removed. Give internally fifteen drops of the SPECIFIC for INFLAMMATION, A A, each morning and night.

In long-standing cases a dose of the SPECIFIC for ULCERS, I I, repeated every few nights will be found of great value, while the A A is given each morning.

Fits, Convulsions, Epilepsy.

The symptoms of fits are pretty well known. Without any or very trifling warning the beast staggers and falls suddenly to the ground; he often bellows in the most alarming manner; then every part of the body is violently convulsed; the tail is lashed; the teeth are ground; the mouth closed, and jaws fastened together; the breathing is quick and attended with heaving at the flanks; frothy slaver dribbles from the mouth, and the urine and dung are discharged involuntarily. In a few moments the convulsions become less severe, then cease, and the animal soon seems as well as if nothing had happened.

Fits are most apt to attack young, vigorous, well-fed cattle, or those that have been much exposed to the direct action of the sun.

TREATMENT.—Little or nothing can be done during an attack; but as one is likely to be followed by another, the medicine should be given as soon as the attack is well over.

Give immediately after the attack twenty drops of the SPECIFIC for CONVULSIONS, A A, and repeat the remedy morning and night for some days.

If an animal is subject to these fits, (epilepsy) returning at intervals of a few days or weeks, give alternately at intervals of six or eight days twenty drops of the SPECIFIC for CONVULSIONS, A A, and that for PARALYSIS, J J, and continue these for some time.

Foul in the Foot, Foot-rot.

Foreign bodies, such as gravel, dirt, stones, etc., especially in moist, low, or marshy places, get into the cleft of the foot, and produce lameness and the following symptoms:

There is lameness and swelling of the pasterns, and heat with evident pain; matter then forms, and unless it is let out, it will extend in all directions under the foot, and appear at the coronet or top of the hoof; and from this long narrow ulcers remain, and proud flesh springs up from the diseased places.

TREATMENT.—Examine the foot carefully, and remove all foreign substances, dirt, etc., that may be found; then foment the foot with hot water night and morning, and afterwards apply THE MARVEL, and wrap it in a turnip or oatmeal poultice; the hoof should be pared, and those parts of it cut away that may interfere with the escape of matter; all dead hoof must be removed. The sore must be examined, and if dark and unhealthy, the MARVEL and poultices must be renewed from time to time until the dark matter sloughs off. After the ulcer looks clean, apply tar and melted tallow in equal proportions, over which tow must be kept wrapped around to prevent dirt lodging in the wound and causing fresh irritation These may be renewed, if needful, until entire recovery.

Give also, the SPECIFIC for ULCERS, I I, each night, a dose of twenty drops.

Mange.

This disease consists of a violent itching and irritation of the surface, and is liable to attack all badly kept domestic animals. It may be caused by overfeeding, or want of wholesome, nutritious food; either extreme may induce it. Thus suddenly changing a cow from a very poor to a rich pasture may induce it, or it may be communicated from one cow to another.

The symptoms are: great itchiness, so that the animal is continually rubbing herself; the hair falls off, scabs or sores remain in patches on the back and tail especially; the cow becomes thin; appetite fails; her milk is reduced in quantity and quality, and she becomes a miserable object.

TREATMENT.—Cleanse the skin by means of a brush, which must not be used for another animal without having been thoroughly washed and cleansed, otherwise it will communicate the disease; afterwards go over again with warm water and soft soap, and carefully dry the surface. Give night and morning twenty drops of the SPECIFIC for ERUPTIONS, I I.

Should the sore spots not readily heal, apply the Sulphur Ointment, or still better the Witch-Hazel oil. (See page 49.)

Hidebound.

This condition, in which the skin seems firm, hard, and bound to the parts beneath, is due to some morbid condition of the system rather than to a disease of the skin itself. There is most frequently some derangement of the stomach, or some old standing organic disease. Remove these, and the disease disappears, and the hide becomes soft and loose.

TREATMENT.—The SPECIFIC for INDIGESTION, ILL CONDITION, J J, giving twenty drops morning and night, will generally remove the difficulty.

If it fails after a fair trial, give the SPECIFIC for INDIGESTION, J J, each night and that for ERUPTION I I, each morning twenty drops.

CHAPTER II.

DISEASES OF THE ORGANS OF RESPIRATION.

Choryza, or Cold in the Head

THIS very common affection consists of an irritation, and sometimes inflammation of the lining membrane of the nose It is usually caused by exposure to cold or wet, or too sudden changes of weather; it is sometimes the commencement of catarrh, and is most frequent during winter and early spring; or it may arise from the irritation of dust inhaled during a long journey.

SYMPTOMS.—In some cases of cold the irritation is confined to the nose alone, and is then known as CHORYZA. It is manifested by a discharge from the nose, first thin and watery, afterward becoming thicker like matter, and corrosive, fretting the skin.

If the disease extends along the air passages, bronchitis or even inflammation of the lungs results, manifested by the cough, fever, and difficulty of breathing peculiar to these affections.

TREATMENT.—For mere choryza or cold in the head, give the SPECIFIC for DISTEMPER, J J, a dose of twenty drops morning and night.

If symptoms of Fever, Bronchitis, or Pneumonia should be present, interpose a few doses of the FEVER SPECIFIC, A A, twenty drops, repeated every three or four hours, which will promptly relieve. Consult also what is said on Bronchitis or Pneumonia.

Hoose, Catarrh, or Common Cold

Differs from the Choryza as the irritation involves the lining membrane of the entire air passages. It is most frequent in the changeable weather of spring and fall, when cattle are exposed to frequent alternations of temperature, or when too many cows are crowded together in a stable, rendering the air hot and impure. Young beasts and cows after calving are especially subject to hoose.

SYMPTOMS.—Dry nose, frequent cough, discharge from the nostrils, stiffness of the limbs, disinclination to move, purging, cold skin, and then hot; imperfect chewing of the cud, failing of milk, watery eyes, quick pulse and breathing. It is very frequent and very fatal in calves, and requires to be attended to promptly in all cases, or it will end in some more dangerous disease.

TREATMENT.—During the earlier stage, with fever, heat, quick pulse and breathing, give the FEVER SPECIFIC, A A, a dose of twenty drops four times per day.

Should cough and irritation remain, or not yield prompty to the FEVER SPECIFIC, give the SPECIFIC E E for COUGH, the same dose, repeated four times daily; or if fever yet continues, give the two SPECIFICS in alternation at intervals of three hours.

For calves, give one-third or half as much as for grown cattle, according to age or size.

Sore Throat or Pharyngitis.

The disease consists of inflammation, with consequent swelling and soreness of the top of the gullet or passage between the mouth and stomach. It arises from the same causes which produce colds, and sometimes assumes an epidemic and very fatal character, especially when the spring or fall is very cold and wet, and the animals graze on damp, marshy grounds. It is usually accompanied with catarrh.

SYMPTOMS.—Difficulty of swallowing, so that solid food is partially chewed and then dropped from the mouth; fluids are gulped down, or partly return through the nostrils; or all food may be refused in consequence of the severe pain attending swallowing; the cud is not chewed; the throat and glands of the neck are swelled, hot, and painful; the cough is frequent, hoarse, and indicates pain; the breathing becomes very difficult and labored, and the pulse full and quick.

TREATMENT.—Give twenty drops of the SPECIFIC for INFLAMMATION, A A, every three or four hours, until three doses have been given, then begin with the SPECIFIC C C, for QUINCY or SORE THROAT, and give every three hours of the C C in alternation with the A A. As the animal improves and the fever and heat abate, the A A may be discontinued, and the C C be used alone at intervals of four or six hours to complete the cure

In all febrile diseases of cattle, it is of the utmost importance to house them in a *warm*, *dry*, *comfortable stable*, free from exposure, dampness, or cold drafts of air, especially in cold or moist weather.

Cough.

Cough in the cow is rarely or never a disease of itself, but merely a symptom or attendant of some disease of the respiratory organs, such as Catarrh, Bronchitis, Pleurisy, or Pneumonia, of which it is merely the indication. Its symptomatic importance is such that it always deserves attention, and its cause should at once be carefully investigated. In some case very grave alterations may be going on in the lungs, which will escape notice if attention be not directed to it by means of the cough. Examine the animal carefully, ascertain the state of her pulse, breathing, appetite, secretion of milk, etc., and direct treatment for such disease as is found to be present.

However, in the absence of any special indications, the SPECIFIC for COUGH, E E, should be given, a dose of twenty drops morning and night, which will generally relieve and will not be out of place in any case.

Bronchitis, or Inflammation of the Bronchial Tubes.

This disease is usually the result of exposure to cold and wet, or sudden changes of temperature; it is almost always preceded by a common cold which has been neglected or overlooked.

SYMPTOMS.—Cough, which becomes by degrees more painful, frequent, and husky; the countenance becomes anxious and distressed; the breathing is quick, heaving, and obstructed, in consequence of tough tenacious phlegm; unwillingness to move; the breath is hot; the cough is increased by moving about, occurs in fits, and is wheezing in character; no food is eaten; the animal wastes; skin becomes dry, and is bound to the ribs; the coat stares and looks unthrifty. The animal may die from extension of the disease to the substance of the lungs, as in "lung disease."

TREATMENT.—The earlier stages of this disease, or catarrh, should be treated at once, as directed under that head. Then a dose or two of the SPECIFIC for that disease removes all danger.

Remove the animal to a warm but well-ventilated stable, and feed on warm mashes and gruel.

Give first, at intervals of two hours, two or three doses of the SPECIFIC for FEVER, A A, twenty drops at a dose. This will allay the heat and fever to some extent. Then alternate at intervals of three hours, the SPECIFIC for COUGH, E E, with that for FEVER, A A, the same doses, and continue this treatment until restored, only that the medicine need not be given so frequently after improvement has progressed.

Pleurisy.

This disease consists of an inflammation of the delicate membrane which lines the chest, and also is reflected over or covers the lungs.

It is caused most frequently by exposure to cold, or from the extension of catarrh. Pleurisy rarely exists alone, but is almost invariably complicated with bronchitis or pneumonia, or both.

SYMPTOMS.—The disease generally begins in the same manner as pneumonia, with dullness, loss of appetite, etc. The cough is attended with pain, and seems to be cut short as if the animal tried to stop it; the breathing is short, seemingly cut off and evidently painful during the passage of the air into the lungs, and is attended with a grunt during its expiration; the sides are painful when pressed upon; the skin, at the angles of the mouth, is wrinkled; the shoulders and upper part of the chest are in a constant quiver; the head is stretched out; the eyes are unusually bright; the tongue hangs out of the mouth, from which frothy slaver is continually flowing. The animal neither eats nor chews the cud; she gets weaker and thinner every day, and all the symptoms become more and more severe until death ensues, often preceded by excessive purging.

TREATMENT.—Give at first the FEVER SPECIFIC, A A, a dose of twenty drops every two hours, and continue this the first day, and night if the case is severe.

Then alternate the SPECIFIC for INFLAMED LUNGS, E E, with that for FEVER, A A, at intervals of two, three, or four hours until the animal is cured.

FOOD AND STABLING.—In all serious diseases of the air-passages, Bronchitis, Pleurisy, Pneumonia, etc., the animal should be placed in a dry, comfortable stable, not too close, and her food should consist of bran-mashes, boiled carrots or turnips, meal-gruel, and hay tea. Good old hay may be given *sparingly;* straw and chaff not at all. When the appetite is returning, great care must be taken not to give too much food at once, for if the stomach is overloaded or crammed, disease is almost sure to return and the animal to die in consequence. *Give but very sparingly of food,* until the stomach has fully regained its former power of digestion.

Pneumonia, or Inflammation of the Lungs.

This is an inflammation of the substance of the lungs, or lights, and is rarely unaccompanied with pleurisy or bronchitis. It is usually brought on by exposure to cold or sudden changes of temperature, or from the extension of a common cold.

The SYMPTOMS are as follows: The cow becomes dull, disinclined to move, and hangs her head; the muzzle is dry; the mouth hot; the cough frequent and dry; the coat rough and staring; the horns, ears, and feet are hot at one time and cold at another; the breathing is quickened and attended with heaving of the flanks; the pulse is full and quick; appetite is gone, and chewing of the cud suspended. The thirst is great, bowels bound and dung dark-colored, the spine is tender when pressed upon, the head projected forward and eyes staring; tears flow down the face; the teeth are ground; a discharge flows from the nose, at first clear and watery, afterwards red and containing some blood; the breathing becomes quicker, more difficult, and labored as the disease advances; the cough comes on in fits; the nostrils are widened, and play to their utmost limit; the body is covered with sweat; the pulse becomes weaker and increased in frequency, and these symptoms increase in violence and become gradually worse until the animal dies.

TREATMENT.—Give, the first twelve or twenty-four hours, the SPECIFIC for FEVER, A A, a dose of twenty drops every two hours.

After the fever and heat have been thus in a measure subdued, alternate the SPECIFIC for INFLAMED LUNGS, E E, with that for FEVER, A A, at intervals of three hours, giving as before twenty drops at a dose.

Continue this treatment steadily, except that unless the case is very critical and urgent, the medicine need not to be kept up during the night, but a dose of the SPECIFIC, E E, may be given late in the night and be permitted to act undisturbed until the morning; then go on as before.

For food and stabling, consult the article on Pleurisy, page 191.

Pleuro-Pneumonia, Pulmonary Murrain, Lung Disease.

This disease is not at this time a frequent one in the United States, at least, in its more violent or epidemic form. But in Europe and the British Isles, it has been known for many years, and has at times raged there as well as here as a most destructive and fatal epizootic, sweeping off a large portion of the stock on a farm, destroying almost every animal attacked. Old school treatment has met it and tried its resources upon it with much the same results as it has met the cholera or similar new diseases; and after having assiduously purged, violently blistered and setoned its patients, and tried all its arts upon them, has only seen the victims die a little quicker under this treatment than without any at all. So much so, that the belief obtains among very many cow keepers that the disease is utterly incurable.

Within the past few years it has made its appearance in various sections of this country, said to have been imported from Holland, and has occasionally made sad ravages among the best imported stock of the vicinity. Within a few short months it extended in various directions from its first locality, overleaping all precautionary measures essayed for its arrest and removal. The attempt to stay its progress by a sanitary cordon, and the indiscriminate slaughter of all animals tainted or suspected, though proper in themselves in reasonable limits, failed, as all such attempts have failed in regard to cholera and similar diseases The English government have, however, succeeded, in thus "stamping out" the disease for a time at least. Such invasions are best subdued when their true homeopathic treatment is understood, and the preventive measures suggested by the law of *similia* applied. That this will be the experience in regard to this new enemy we do not hesitate to affirm. According to all experience it will prevail more or less extensively in this country, and hence it is well to be acquainted with its symptoms and treatment.

Homeopathy has been very successful in subduing this disease, and we are assured, from repeated trials, that all animals may be saved that are treated in the earlier stages, and even a fair proportion of the extreme cases.

CAUSES.—The causes of such forms of disease are involved in obscurity, but it is wel' known that certain circumstances strongly pre dispose to its development. These are: low, damp, badly ventilated, ill-drained stables; swampy, damp, boggy districts, in which there is a great decomposition of vegetable matter. It usually prevails at certain seasons of the year, and is most common in the late fall and early spring, or during damp chilly weather. Some animals are more liable to attack than others; it is not so frequent and is more manageable in the open country than in extensive close stables in large towns, where animals are crowded together, live an unnatural life, and are milked very dry in order to increase the daily yield. Many persons suppose it to arise from some atmospheric condition similar to that of cholera, and it is generally considered contagious, that is, communicated from diseased to healthy cows by contact or immediate contiguity.

SYMPTOMS.—These have been found to vary in different epidemics and seasons, nor does every animal attacked present all the symptoms of the entire disease. Yet, taking several animals together, the complete picture of the disease will be found, and each animal will also present sufficient characteristic symptoms to identify the malady. In the first stage the attack has been known to vary, thus: the attack coming on with great violence, and running a rapid course in spite of all treatment; or, it may come on slowly and insidiously, the animal not seeming very ill until her lungs are diseased beyond all hope of recovery; or, it may announce itself with violent purging, great weakness, and rapid loss of flesh.

The majority of cases, however, present the following symptoms: a short, dry, husky cough which is heard only occasionally, and which is highly characteristic of the disease, and when once heard will rarely be mistaken again. The owner says, perhaps, he has heard this "hoose" for two or three days, but has paid no attention to it. On inquiry, we find the animal does not give so much milk as usual, and that it has a slightly yellowish tinge; the appetite is not much imparied, yet she is careless of her food and does not lick her dish clean; when at rest the breathing does not show any departure from its healthy play, but if the animal is moved about or walks some distance, it becomes more frequent, labored, and difficult; the pulse is often healthy in character, although sometimes it is weak and slightly increased in frequency; the bowels may be confined or purged or quite regular; the body is sometimes hot, sometimes cold. The cow appears dull and listless, and when at grass, separates herself from her companions, and lies on the ground when they are feeding.

In the Second Stage.—The cough is now more frequent, and thick frothy phlegm dribbles from the mouth; the breathing is short when the air is taken into the lungs, and long when it is pressed out of them; the inhalation is attended with much pain, causing the animal to grunt and grate her teeth; the grunt is heard when the animal is pressing the air out from her lungs; the pain is evidently increased by coughing and change of position, and to lessen it the cough is now suppressed or held back, and is short, and the cow stands fixed in one place. The pain is owing to the pleura being inflamed, and the inflamed place may be ascertained by pressing the side along between the ribs with the point of the finger, when the animal will flinch and grunt at the diseased place. The pulse becomes quickened and oppressed; the skin hard, tight, and bound to the ribs; the horns are hotter and the muzzle drier than usual; the head is lowered and thrust forward, with the nose poked out; the back is raised up sometimes; little or no food is eaten; the cud is seldom or never chewed; the milk is arrested; bowels are bound, and when moved, the dung is in hard dry lumps.

In the third stage.—The breathing is much more quickened, very difficult, labored, and even gasping; the breathing is carried on partly through the mouth, partly through the nose; the breath has a bad smell; a stringy frothy fluid constantly dribbles from the mouth; the cow groans loudly and frequently while the grunt is either gone or subdued; the pulse is quick weak, and, in some cases, intermittent or even imperceptible; the horns, ears, and legs are cold, the skin covered with cold sweat, the head and neck stretched out, and the nose poked into the corner of the manger; the fore-legs are separated from each other, and fixed in one place, unless the cow is restless and uneasy; sometimes the hind ones are crossed over each other, or the hind fetlock-joints are knuckled forward; the animal is thin and reduced to a skeleton; the strength of course greatly impaired, so that she can scarcely cough; the urine is very high-colored; toward the last, violent purging comes on, the discharged matter being quite watery, blackish, highly offensive, and sometimes mixed with blood; eventually, the cavity of the chest becomes so full of fluid or so much of the lung is condensed, that the breathing, from being more and more difficult, and labored, and frequent, at last ceases, and the animal is dead.

TREATMENT.—Preventive Measures: During the prevalence of such a disease unusual care should be taken of all animals liable to it; for although a contagion may be in the atmosphere or conveyed by contact, yet some untoward circumstance, such as cold, a chill, exposure, or bad food or ventilation, always provokes the attack; hence, at such times especial care should be exercised that food, housing and general management should be unexceptionable.

Give, also, an exposed animal the SPECIFIC for INFLAMED LUNGS, E E, a dose of fifteen drops every night or every second night, experience having abundantly shown that *the Specific for a disease always acts as a preventive when given before the attack.* Medicines, if specific and thus given, are as surely protective as is vaccination a preventive of small-pox.

At the first indications of the disease, the "hoose," which may be a day or two before any other symptoms, give the SPECIFIC for COUGH, E E, and repeat it three times per day, a dose of twenty drops, and the disease will go no farther.

Should the disease have manifested itself with some violence, cough, breathing more or less labored and painful, manifested with the grunt, give the SPECIFIC for FEVER, A A, twenty drops every two hours for twelve hours, and then alternate it with the SPECIFIC for INFLAMED LUNGS, E E. at intervals of two or three hours.

In the fully developed cases of the disease (in the more advanced stages), when there is less *heat* and *fever*, but great weakness, wheezing, short, difficult breathing, small, quick, weak pulse, cold clammy sweats, cold extremities, or with violent purging of blackish offensive matter, omit the FEVER SPECIFIC, A A, and give instead every two hours, first the SPECIFIC for INFLAMED LUNGS, E E, a dose of twenty drops, and the next two hours the SPECIFIC, I I, for ULCERATIONS, a dose of twenty drops, and thus continue the two remedies alternately at intervals of two or three hours. This is the treatment for all the more advanced, confirmed, or malignant forms of this disease, the one remedy corresponding to the local affection of the lung and pleura and the other to the malignant and septic character of the general affection.

The existence of dark, fetid and bloody discharges is no contra-indication for the use of these Specifics, which are fully adapted to that condition.

Food and stabling should be carefully directed, as under the article on Pleurisy, page 191.

Diseased cattle should at once be removed from the healthy stock, and be housed by themselves at some distance from the rest of the herd. The stable should be dry and well ventilated; air and light should be freely admitted, although all draughts of air are highly injurious, and must be guarded against.

CHAPTER III.

DISEASES OF THE ORGANS OF DIGESTION.

Loss of the Cud.

THIS is a mere symptom which accompanies many diseases, and even morbid conditions, which scarcely deserve the name of disease, and will yield with the removal of the ailment of which it is a mere symptom. Sometimes it may be present when nothing else is sufficiently tangible to warrant treatment, or it may continue after the disease otherwise seems to have been removed.

TREATMENT.—In any case in which it appears to exist independently, or to be the principal symptom, give twenty drops of the SPECIFIC for INDIGESTION, J J, morning and night. The "cud" will soon return.

Colic.

This disease is not so dangerous as tympanitis, yet it may prove fatal from bad treatment or neglect. It is generally the result of improper or indigestible food, or food in too great quantity, or that to which the animal is not accustomed. If colic comes on after indigestible food, it is accompanied by constipation and thirst. Certain kinds of food, such as grains, oats, decayed turnips or cabbages, or dry food, are liable to induce it, or it may arise from exposure to cold, when the body is warm, or from cold drinking when the body is heated.

SYMPTOMS.—Sudden manifestation of pain in the belly, by uneasiness, pawing the ground, striking the belly with the hind legs or horns, often lying down and then rising, grinding the teeth, and moaning. When caused by wind, the belly is much swelled on the left side; and there is frequent passage of flatus. The animal's back is arched, and she frequently looks at her flanks, scrapes with her fore-feet, and kicks with the hind ones. All these symptoms increase, until she expires amid groans and grinding of the teeth.

TREATMENT.—The SPECIFIC for COLIC, F F, will almost invariably be found successful. Give a dose of twenty drops every half hour until relieved. If not better after a few doses, and should there be fever, alternate the SPECIFIC, A A, for FEVER, the same dose with that for COLIC, F F, at the same intervals. As the animal seems relieved, or partially so, give the remedies at longer intervals.

Constipation.

This is rarely of grave consequence in cattle, and when it exists, is usually a symptom of some other disease. When present, a dose of twenty drops of the SPECIFIC for INDIGESTION, J J, given morning and night, will soon set all right again. If there is suspicion of some inflammatory condition lurking in the system, the FEVER SPECIFIC, A A, in like doses will have the like effect.

Hoove or Blown, Over-fed.

The most frequent cause is turning an animal into rich pasture, when, from over-eating, the stomach becomes so distended as not to be able to act upon its contents. The food then undergoes chemical changes, in the process of which an immense amount of gas or wind is generated, producing swelling, distension, etc.; drinking very cold water, and especially eating too much bran, chaff, grains, oats, wheat, corn, is followed by similar consequences, in an intensified degree.

SYMPTOMS.—The disease is known by the animal being swelled, or "blown" over the whole belly, but espec ally at the stomach and left side, where the distended stomach lies; the swelling yields to the finger, and gives a hollow drum-like sound when struck; there are sour or noisome belchings of wind; the cow does not move, moans and breathes with difficulty, neither eats nor chews the cud.

As the disease progresses, the pulse becomes full and hard, and quicker than before; the eyes are red and protruded; the mouth is filled with frothy slaver, and the tongue hangs out; the back is crouched, and legs drawn under the body; the cow becomes insensible when the swelling is at its height; she stands in one place, continually moaning or grunting; she falls and struggles violently; sour fluid mixed with food rises from the stomach, and is discharged from her nostrils and mouth, and at last death.

TREATMENT.—Give the SPECIFIC for COLIC, F F, every fifteen minutes, a dose of twenty drops. After an hour, alternate it with the SPECIFIC for INDIGESTION, J J, at the same intervals; and when better, prolong the intervals to half an hour, an hour, or two hours.

In some extreme cases, when, as from eating new clover, or other rank succulent food, the production of gas is immense and the animal rapidly growing worse, the trocar or even a narrow-bladed knife may be used, to afford immediate relief. It must be plunged inward and downward into the paunch, on the left side of the belly, midway between the last rib and the haunch-bone. This is only a resource in extremity, as the SPECIFICS, F F, and J J, in all such cases act promptly and perfectly, as experience has abundantly testified.

Diarrhea, Scouring.

Diarrhea is more common in old cattle and calves than in those of middle age, where it is generally of little importance, soon correcting itself, especially in the spring, when herds are first turned into green fields. The usual causes are, decayed cabbages, bad grains, or other improper food or impure water; sudden change to rich pastures; the use of purgative medicines; exposure to cold and wet; acrid bile;

sudden change from dry to wet weather, or severe exertion in hot dry weather.

SYMPTOMS.—The disease comes on slowly with staring coat, shaking, arched back, fore-legs drawn together, cold legs, ears, and horns, weak pulse, tucked up belly, bowels rather looser than usual, deficient appetite. The animal becomes thinner, more depressed and dull; little or no milk is given, and the bowels are purged to an alarming extent. This purging may stop, and then reappear to end fatally, or terminate in dysentery.

TREATMENT.—We should, of course, give food not so loosening in its character, and the SPECIFIC for DIARRHEA, F F, a dose of twenty drops, two or three times per day, will usually be found quite sufficient. In extreme cases, or in case of failure with this remedy, the SPECIFIC for ULCERS, I I, may be alternated with it, at the same or even more frequent intervals.

Diarrhea, or Skit in Calves.

This disease is quite common, and sometimes dangerous. It may be produced by sudden change of food, too much or too little food, or from some peculiarity in the mother's milk. It may sometimes be the natural means of throwing off something that is injurious to the calf, and hence it would be improper to arrest it. Only when the animal becomes weak, is off its food, does not chew the cud, when there are pains in the belly, or the dung is slimy or mixed with blood, or the discharge is like cream, with wasting of the body, are we imperatively called upon to interfere.

TREATMENT.—Give five or eight drops of the SPECIFIC for DIARRHEA, F F, two or three times per day. If it does not yield promptly, interpose a dose or two of the SPECIFIC for ULCERS, I I, between the others.

Food.—No green food, but gruel of flour or starch, or cooked milk.

Dysentery, Bloody Flux.

This is a very severe and often fatal form of disease, which prevails mostly in spring and fall, and in some sections of country, and in peculiar states of the weather and growth of feed becomes a most destructive scourge. It is usually attributed to feed growing upon wet or marshy grounds, or pasture sometimes under water; or to rank grass growing in the woods; or drink from impure, still, and stagnant waters. It appears also when animals are exposed to alternations of hot and cold weather, live upon bad food, or are over-driven. It is seen in cattle driven a long distance, and insufficiently or badly fed, or with food to which they are not accustomed. Poor and fat cattle are alike subject to it; it comes on after "hoose," or the disappearance of some skin disease, or sudden stoppage of milk, or as a termination of diarrhea.

SYMPTOMS—Shaking, dullness, anxiety, dry skin, slightly rough hair, and general uneasiness. In some cases the bowels seem bound, the dung hard, dry, in small lumps, and the discharge attended with pain; in others the dung is soft, discharged frequently, and the animal wastes, and loses appetite and spirits. In others again, the purging is almost constant, attended with pain, gripes, straining, and forcing out of the fundament. In this stage the discharge is watery, mixed with white shreds, or dark colored blood, with little or no dung, and attended with a horrible bad smell. These violent symptoms may disappear, but the purging and wasting continue as bad as ever, or stop for a short time, and then return again, and continue until the animal is worn out by the constant drain; or, the dysenteric discharges are arrested and improvement begins and goes on slowly. In some extreme cases, the wasting is so excessive that the animal is reduced to a mere bag of bones, the joints swelled, body covered with sores, strength gone, eyes hollow and dim, parts under the jaw enlarged, body covered with vermin, discharges mixed with blood, and horribly offensive, and the skin bedewed with cold sweat. Such extreme cases are often hopeless.

TREATMENT.—Give twenty drops of the SPECIFIC for DYSENTERY, F F, every three hours, or even more frequently in the more urgent cases.

In the extreme cases, with great prostration and weakness, alternate the SPECIFIC for ULCERS, I I, with that for DYSENTERY, F F, at intervals of two or three hours, and continue the course patiently, prolonging the intervals between the doses as the animal improves.

Irregular Teeth

May be looked for if an animal presents the following symptoms: The beast becoming thinner gradually, and eating less food than usual; slaver dribbling from the mouth along with half chewed food, especially while the cow is cudding; she is "hoven" or bloated at different times; a bad smell comes from the mouth, arising from ulceration of the side of the cheek, caused by irregular teeth.

TREATMENT.—The mouth must be carefully examined, and all long or irregular teeth must be shortened and smoothed by means of the tooth-rasp.

Jaundice, the Yellows.

This may be caused by torpidity of the liver itself, or obstruction of the gall-duct, in consequence of hardened bile (gall-stones) filling up the passage, or from the presence of the fluke-worm in the gall-duct; or it may arise from inflammation or other disease of the liver.

SYMPTOMS.—These will vary from the progress and severity of the disease and the causes which produce it, but it will essentially be as follows: In some cases the pulse is full, hard and accelerated; the breathing quickened, with panting at the flanks, thirst, hot mouth, scanty urine, loss of cud and appetite, and other symptoms of fever. In some cases there is loss of spirits, dullness, or sleepiness, unwillingness to move, and weakness; the body wastes and shows other signs of impaired condition; the eyes, skin and urine are at first tinged with yellow, which afterward becomes deeper and more distinct; scales form on the skin; the bowels are at first confined, but purging afterward comes on, and may be so rapid and excessive that it can not be arrested, and the animal dies in consequence. The milk also becomes yellowish and somewhat bitter.

TREATMENT.—The SPECIFIC for JAUNDICE, J J, may be given, twenty drops morning and night, in the torpid cases when there is little or no fever. But when fever and hot mouth are present alternate the SPECIFIC for FEVER, A A, with that for JAUNDICE, J J, four times per day in the same doses, that is two doses of each during the day.

If a violent purging comes on give twenty drops of the SPECIFIC for DIARRHEA, F F, every three hours until relieved, and then return to the SPECIFIC for JAUNDICE, J J.

Hepatitis, Inflammation of the Liver.

This disease is more common in oxen than in horses. It is rarely seen except in winter, and in animals fed in the stable. It may be mistaken for inflammation of the chest, to which it has some resemblance.

SYMPTOMS.—The animal prefers lying down, but always on the left side, and with the head turned to the right. The heat is greater in the region of the liver on the right side, and pressure there induces pain; the animal eats little or nothing, and can not walk or stand up without pain, constantly stumbling. If the disease is acute there is high fever, with increased heat of body and accelerated pulse; the horns and ears are alternately hot and cold; the milk is yellowish and bitter, portions of the skin are denuded of hair; the eyes, mouth, gums, and tongue (which are covered with thick mucus), the nose and teats are *yellow*; the urine is of deep yellow color; and there is sometimes a dry and painful cough. In chronic hepatitis the fever is considerable or wanting altogether, but the yellow tint is more marked and general; the milk equally yellow and bitter, soon forms a caseous mass, from which a yellow serum separates; the right side of the body seems tense and swollen; the intestines do not empty themselves, or the scanty ejections resemble putty or clay. The acute form lasts from eight to fifteen days, and the chronic many months.

TREATMENT.—In the more acute form, attended with heat and fever, the SPECIFIC for FEVER, A A, should be given; a dose of twenty drops four times per day.

In the chronic form the SPECIFIC, A A, may be given each morning, and that for INDIGESTION J J, each evening, twenty drops, which will usually be found sufficient.

Gloss Anthrax, Blain, Black Tongue.

This is an epidemic, and sometimes fearfully fatal disease, which has prevailed under different modifications at various seasons, in different sections of the country. It appears to have its origin in some peculiar atmospheric conditions, favored doubtless by exposure or impoverished keeping, and is then propagated from diseased to healthy animals. It is most common in spring and fall.

SYMPTOMS.—The animal appears low-spirited dull and does not eat or chew the cud; a clear fluid without smell, constantly flows from the mouth; the head and neck constantly swell, until they are much increased in size; the breathing becomes difficult and obstructed, in some cases so much so that the animal cannot breathe, and death results early from suffocation; the fluid from the mouth becomes like matter, or is mixed with blood, and of very disagreeable odor; the tongue becomes swollen, and its sides covered with large, red blisters, which rapidly increase in size, and at last burst, discharging their contents, and leaving deep sores, which are apt to mortify. Other blisters successively arise, and run the same course. Symptoms of low fever come on, the whole of the tongue becomes inflamed and swelled; at last a portion of it mortifies, turns black, and the animal dies, sometimes within a few hours from the beginning of the disease.

TREATMENT.—The diseased animal must be removed from the herd, and care be taken to prevent healthy animals being affected, by not using the same vessels or articles for both. The attendant should be careful not to get the fluid from the mouth upon any sore on the hand or person, or he will be likely to suffer. The blisters forming on the tongue or mouth of the animal should be opened freely as early as possible

Food—As the cow cannot swallow, on account of the pain and swelling of the tongue, gruel should be horned down occasionally during the day. Some should also be placed before her, so that she may take it if she feels disposed.

Give the SPECIFIC for DISTEMPER, C C, a dose of twenty or twenty-five drops, every one, two, or three hours, according to the intensity of the disease. After twelve hours, or three or four doses have been given, if the animal does not seem to improve, give the SPECIFIC I I, in doses of twenty drops, in alternation with the C C, at intervals of two or three hours, and so continue through the entire disease.

Splenitis, or Inflammation of the Spleen.

Splenitis is rarely observed in oxen except in cold' damp weather, and it differs from carbuncle or typhus, but occasions death no less rapidly. Its prominent symptom is a *brownish color of the tongue.* It is most frequent among working cattle, especially if put to labor soon after eating, and before they have had time to chew the cud.

SYMPTOMS.—It generally begins with symptoms of pain in the belly, attended with quickened breathing and heaving at the flanks; pain is manifested at the upper part of the flanks when pressed upon; the muzzle is dry and roughened, and the tongue brownish; there are frequent low moanings; no appetite or chewing of the cud; a swelling will be found at the left side and flank, which may be mistaken for hoove; but the two diseases will be distinguished by noticing that in hoove the swelling is greater and comes on very rapidly, and that when struck upon a clear, hollow, drum-like sound is returned, while in inflammation of the spleen the sound is dull and heavy; the animal is lame when he walks, or he walks with difficulty.

TREATMENT.—The SPECIFIC for FEVER, A A, will be found to cover the disease perfectly. Give twenty drops every four hours.

CHAPTER IV.

DISEASES OF THE URINARY AND GENITAL ORGANS.

Dropping after calving; milk fever; puerperal fever.

THIS disease is of frequent occurrence and quite liable to be fatal, unless under proper homeopathic treatment. It is much more prevalent some seasons than others, owing, doubtless, to peculiar atmospheric conditions, and is more malignant some seasons than others. The ordinary methods of treatment, purging and bleeding, etc., does more harm than good, and few cows survive the double infliction of dosing and disease combined. The proper use of the Homeopathic Specifics, however, rarely fails to restore even in the worst cases.

There are certain causes which predispose to this disease; thus, fat, stall-fed cows are more liable to it than poor or lean ones; the complaint is more common in the variable weather of early spring and late fall; a cow once having the disease is more liable to a return than others. The exciting causes are: exposure to cold and wet; driving the cow a long journey too soon; giving too much or too rich food soon after calving.

SYMPTOMS.—This fever begins shortly after calving, usually within twenty-four hours; if three or four days pass over, the cow may be considered safe from an attack. The earlier symptoms are: the cow refuses her food or only eats a little of it; she is depressed, hangs her head and looks dull; the horns are hot; the nose, instead of being damp with healthy dew, becomes hot and dry; the urine is scanty; the bowels are confined, or, if moved, the dung is hard and lumpy; the pulse is quicker and fuller than in health; the breathing is quickened and attended with heaving at the flanks.

To these warning symptoms are added with more or less rapidity, the more formidable ones which are often first to attract the attention of the owner. The milk is reduced in quantity or entirely stopped; the eyes glisten and look bright and staring; the white of the eye is covered with numerous red streaks, or is of a leaden color; the eye balls are thrust forward in their sockets, and give the cow a somewhat wild and anxious expression; the hind legs seem weak, and are separated a little from each other; she appears to stand uneasily upon them, resting for a time on one foot and then changing to the other; this paddling and shifting from one leg to another continues as the difficulty of standing increases until the animal supports herself by leaning against the stall; she does not chew the cud; all discharge from the bearing is stopped; the calf is neglected; the pulse becomes slower than before, and the breathing more difficult; the udder is hard and swelled, and little or no milk can be drawn from it; gradually becoming worse, the weakness in the hind-legs increases, so they can no longer support her; she staggers and sways about, falling at length heavily on the ground; she struggles, tries to rise again, and may or may not succeed, but in either case soon loses the power of rising, and lies helpless upon the ground. In this stage of the complaint the symptoms vary. In some cases we have the following: the cow tosses her head from side to side, writhes her body, and lashes her tail, struggles, stretches out her hind-legs, moans and bellows and seems to suffer great pain. The breathing is also difficult and labored; the skin covered with clammy sweat; the paunch enormously swollen from accumulated gas. Unless this swelling subsides, the breathing becomes more difficult and labored; the pulse more rapid and oppressed, so as scarcely to be counted; the legs very cold; pain is worse; fetid gas rises from the stomach, and death ensues.

In other cases the foregoing symptoms are absent, or exist only in a slight degree; and we have the following: The cow lies stretched out at full length on her side, or her head is brought to the opposite side, with the nose towards the shoulder, and the chin on the ground; or the head is twisted directly backward, with the nose held out, and the horns upon the shoulder, in the most awkward manner. The eyes are dim and glassy; the pupils are dilated, rounded, and do not contract at the approach of light; the ears drop, the mouth is partly open; the lower jaw drops if the head is raised; she has not the power to hold up the head; she has lost the sense of feeling, and can scarcely swallow, if at all; difficult, rattling breathing; pulse weak, slow, and intermittent, or even imperceptible; horns, legs, and surface cold and chilly; swelling of the belly increases; udder swelled, hard, and sometimes red on the outside; in some cases dung and urine suppressed. All these symptoms become worse by degrees, and unless relieved, death ensues generally within two days from the attack, sometimes in a few hours.

TREATMENT.—The symptoms of this disease appear so suddenly, and run so rapid a course, that if the disease is prevailing, or there is reason from any cause to apprehend it, the cow should be watched about the time of calving, and a dose or two of fifteen drops of the FEVER SPECIFIC, A A, should be given soon after. This will act as a preventive and arrest any premonitions of the disease, and we would counsel its continuance; at least an occasional dose morning and night for two or three days. It will favor the early and feverless production of milk, and prevent the formation of fever.

Should the disease have made its appearance with evident fever, unequal warmth, bloating, suppressed discharge from the bearing, etc., give the SPECIFIC for FEVER, A A, a dose of twenty drops every two or three hours until the disease is arrested. This remedy is the appropriate specific for all the stages and forms of this disease, and requires only its faithful employment to relieve and cure even the most formidable cases.

Only in the last extremity, with labored breathing, extreme bloating, and entire loss or rapid failure of strength, the SPECIFIC for ULCERS, I I, may be alternated with the FEVER SPECIFIC, A A, at intervals of two hours in doses of twenty drops until the system rallies, when the two medicines may be continued at longer intervals

NURSING AND CARE.—The cow should be placed in a clean, roomy stall, so as to be allowed to rise and to be attended with facility; laid on clean, dry straw, no dung allowed to remain, and be comfortably clothed according to the season. The milk should be frequently drawn off and the udder hand-rubbed. She should lie with the fore part of her body higher than the hinder part, or on a level, with her legs under her in a natural position. She must be on her side and supported by bundles of straw, and on no account be allowed to lie out full stretched, in which position she will become worse and surely die. Small quantities of warm gruel are best for food.

Abortion or Slinking.

The natural period of calving is two hundred and eighty-five days after conception; if it occurs before this period it is termed an abortion. A cow is most liable to abort between the fifth and eighth month. At some seasons, from causes not fully explained, but supposed to be atmospheric, cows are very liable to slink their calves, and when it occurs in a herd it is very liable to extend to others, and may become very general unless proper measures are taken to arrest it.

Aside from the endemic or epidemic causes adverted to, the more common occasions of slinking are: Blows, falls, strains, severe exertions, and injuries, or other forcible or violent movements; severe illness, such as consumption, hoove, inflammation of the bowels, especially if caused by eating grass covered with hoar frost; eating herbs which grow in low marshy places; drinking water impregnated with iron; intercourse with the bull during pregnancy; exposure to foul smells arising from decayed animal matter, especially if it be the cleansing of a cow that has just slunk; over-fed cows are more liable to miscarry than those in moderate condition; suddenly placing a lean, starved cow upon a rich pasture, or a fat cow upon poor food; fright may produce it. A cow who has once aborted is almost certain to do so again.

SYMPTOMS.—The indications which should warn an owner that his cow is about to miscarry are often unnoticed, unless he is particularly observing. They are as follows: Dullness; loss of spirits; want of appetite; loss of cud; more or less completely arrested secretion of milk; hollow flanks; enlargement of the lower part of the belly; staggering whilst walking; disinclination to move, both when standing up and when lying down; the movements of the calf, previously vigorous, become less frequent, and soon cease; the breathing is labored and quickened; a yellowish discharge comes from the bearing; the belly continues to fall; the cow is feverish and moans occasionally; the calf-bed contracts at last and expels the calf, which is usually dead, or dies in a short time.

TREATMENT.—The cow should be placed by herself in a well-aired, quiet stable; food should be light and sloppy; fat cows should not be fed on rich and stimulating food, while lean ones should receive that which is more nourishing. If the calf is dead, the sooner it passes off the better; and it should be deeply buried away from the cattle or herd.

Give fifteen drops of the SPECIFIC for MISCARRIAGE, G G, every six hours, and the dose may be repeated two or three times should the threatening symptoms continue after the first or even second dose has expended its action.

This interval should elapse between doses, as too rapid ones may even defeat the object, by over-excitement of the system, while a single dose often arrests a miscarriage at once.

If a cow has previously miscarried, she should have every few days along about the time when it may be expected, a dose of the above SPECIFIC as a preventive; or if slinking prevails in a herd or neighborhood, a dose of the SPECIFIC for MISCAR-

RIAGE, G G, given once or twice per week, will arrest its progress and prevent miscarriage, a result that can only be achieved by this benign and scientific treatment.

Cleaning after Calving.

In some cases, from torpidity of the calf-bed, the afterbirth is retained, which may result in very serious consequences.

A dose of twenty drops of the SPECIFIC for MISCARRIAGE, G G, will soon cause its expulsion and the healthy cleaning of the animal. It may be repeated at intervals of four hours, if necessary.

Flooding after Calving.

Some blood is necessarily lost after calving, and it is only when the amount is excessive or continues some time, or threatens to weaken or destroy the animal, that the term flooding can be applied to it. It may be occasioned by injuries received during the process of delivery, or from the calf-bed not sufficiently contracting from atony or want of vigor of that organ.

The symptoms need not be described; any continuous flowing from the bearing, before or after delivery, and especially after the passage of the cleansing, should receive medication.

TREATMENT.—The cow should be kept quiet and be permitted to lie down, and twenty drops of the SPECIFIC for HEMORRHAGE, G G, be given every hour, or even every half-hour in urgent cases.

Cold injections, cold wet cloths applied to the loins, or cold water poured upon the belly, are not necessary, and are not without danger.

Sore Teats.

The teats crack into sores, which become painful, and discharge, the contents mingling with the milk; the pain occasioned during milking renders the cow restive, and soon tends to make her vicious and to keep back her milk; garget hence is apt to arise from the milk remaining in the udder and causing irritation.

TREATMENT.—The majority of the cases will be rapidly cured by washing them carefully and gently with warm water, morning and night, and then bathe them with THE MARVEL, or yet better anointing them with the WITCH HAZEL-OIL giving, also, morning and night, fifteen drops of the SPECIFIC for ULCERS, I I. Great care should also be taken to perfectly empty the udder at each milking. If not better after five or six days, use the. SPECIFIC, J J, instead.

Garget, or Inflammation of the Udder.

This is most liable to arise after the first calving, and may be traced to exposure to cold and damp, especially if the cow is in good condition, or from not milking the cow clean, so that the milk remains and causes irritation, or in some cases, the bag may be wounded by lying upon it.

SYMPTOMS.—A portion of the bag becomes hot, painful, and swollen; then little hard lumps can be felt in the teats or in one quarter of the bag; other parts of it become affected in the same way; the pulse is full, quick, and hard; breathing is quickened; the mouth and horns hot; bowels bound, and other symptoms of fever are present. If the disease is allowed to go on. the fever becomes more severe; the cow does not eat or chew the cud; the swelling, previously hard, becomes soft from the formation of matter; the milk becomes mixed with matter, and in some cases, with blood. If the matter is not let out, it will spread through the bag, making its way slowly to the skin, through which it at last bursts, leaving deep long ulcers, which heal with difficulty, and in many cases a portion of the udder is lost, as regards its power to produce milk. If this result is avoided by judicious treatment, some hardness may remain which requires time to remove.

TREATMENT.—Keep the udder well milked out, and give the SPECIFIC for FEVER, A A, twenty drops four times per day. This will generally disperse the heat, hardness, and inflammation. But should suppuration have come on and the abscess point or show a soft spot, lance it, and then give the SPECIFIC for ULCERS, I I, morning and night, until healed.

Red Water.

This disease is most common in spring and fall, and most frequent in low, damp places; it may be brought on by eating certain medicinal plants or by drinking impure water; sudden changes of weather, or disorders of the stomach and liver, or change of pasture, sometimes induce it, and it is not unfrequent after calving.

SYMPTOMS.--The earlier symptoms, such as dullness, loss of appetite, staring coat, dry nose, and tender loins, may not be observed, and the color of the urine may be the first thing to attract attention or indicate the nature of the complaint. The water is at first more or less red; the breathing is quick, labored, and attended with heaving at the flanks; the legs, ears, and horns are cold; the pulse is small and wiry, and the milk is of a reddish hue. As the disease advances, the urine increases in redness, and towards the last becomes yellowish and then quite black; the pulse becomes weak; the white of the eye, and every part of the skin that can be seen, are of a brownish yellow color, the animal gradually loses strength and flesh, the eyes are sunken in their sockets, and at last death ensues, preceded in some cases, by excessive purging.

TREATMENT.—Give the SPECIFIC for FEVER, A A, a dose of twenty drops three or four times per day.

Should the disease not yield within two or three days, the FEVER SPECIFIC may be alternated with that for SCANTY URINATION, H H, twenty drops four times per day. The first mentioned SPECIFIC will, however, generally be found sufficient.

Suppressed or Scanty Urination.

This is usually the result of some disease of the kidneys or a mere symptom of other morbid condition, or it may arise from a paralytic condition of the bladder itself. This condition will generally be promptly relieved by giving a few doses of the SPECIFIC for SCANTY or SUPPRESSED URINATION, H H, twenty drops at intervals of four, six, or twelve hours, according to the urgency of the case.

Inflammation of the Bladder, Cystitis.

This disease is not so common in cattle as in horses, but may be occasioned by cold or injuries in the region of the loins. It is manifested by the following—

SYMPTOMS.—The animal constantly keeps the back arched; the walk is stiff, and the animal when standing leans against something on one side or the other; frequent effort to pass water, but to little purpose, as only a small quantity, of deep red color, is passed at a time. The bowels are bound, evacuations scanty, and passed with pain. There is no appetite or rumination, but intense thirst; the eyes are prominent and the countenance evinces great distress.

TREATMENT. The SPECIFIC for INFLAMED BLADDER, H H, will be found perfectly appropriate, and may be repeated in doses of twenty drops every three or four hours, until entire relief is experienced.

Inflammation of the Kidneys, Nephritis.

This disease has many symptoms in common with Cystitis, or Inflammation of the Bladder, and its treatment scarcely differs. It occasionally occurs in cattle, and may be excited by blows upon the loins, calculi, or small stones formed in the kidneys, or by eating poisonous plants, or the use of strong allopathic medicines.

SYMPTOMS.—The animal brings the fore-legs together, bends the back downwards, and presses with pain when endeavoring to pass water; the loins are hot, more so than the remainder of the body, sometimes even burning. The rectum is hot, dung scanty, and passed with pain. There is a great desire to pass water, but only a few drops escape, which is at first limpid, then thick and of a deep red color. The gait is stiff, appetite gone, no rumination, but great thirst.

TREATMENT.—Give the SPECIFIC for INFLAMED KIDNEYS, H H, a dose of twenty drops every two, three, or four hours, according to the intensity of the disease. It will be found entirely sufficient.

Gonorrhea, Bull-Burnt, Clap.

This disease is usually a consequence of diseased organs of the other sex; or it may be induced in a modified degree from want of cleanliness or from the irritation of repeated acts of coition.

If it arises from contact with the diseased organs of the male, it begins to manifest itself in from two to four days after connection, the first symptoms being a peculiar side-motion of the tail, which is otherwise kept rather close over the fundament; the bearing is at first swelled and sore, afterwards much more swollen, separated, and red on the inside; a mattery discharge sometimes in considerable quantities flows out; the urine is small in quantity, made very frequently, and with much pain.

In the male the sheath is red and swelled; a constant discharge of matter issues from it; great pain and scalding attend the act of urinating, and the water is voided in small quantities and in a jerking manner.

TREATMENT.—The prepuce or sheath of the bull, or the bearing of the cow, should be cleansed and kept clean with tepid water and soap; after which the parts may be washed with THE MARVEL, or it may be injected, morning and night. Give three times per day twenty drops of the SPECIFIC for PAINFUL URINATION, H H, and continue its use two or three times per day until cured. The SPECIFIC, H H, will entirely control the disease, yet if time is important we can hasten the cure by means of the MARVEL as above indicated.

PART III.

DISEASES OF SHEEP.

CHAPTER I.

DISEASES OF THE DIGESTIVE SYSTEM.

ANTHRAX FEVER.—Known as *Black-leg; Quarter ill*; or the *Black Spauld* of the English Shepards, of as one of the "Murrains" of this country. It effects young and thrifty sheep, and is rarely found in old and poor stock. It is most common in we seasons, in the early spring, or summer and fall, and when the feed is very luxuriant. The sheep gorge themselves with the rich vegetation, and the diges tion being overtaxed, the system is disorganized and the sheep suddenly droop and die. On examination the wool leaves the skin at the slightest touch. and the body is found to be swollen and blackened in large patches, chiefly on the hind or fore-quarter Air is infiltrated under the skin and the carcas seems already decomposed and full of black blood. On examining the flock, some will be lame or limping, the eyes red, and the mouth and tongue inflamed and blistered, and on passing the hand over the sides on quarters, they will be found swollen, the wool readily coming off, and a crepitation be heard from the confined air beneath. The urine is dark, the bowels constipated and dung bloody. After a time the animal is unable to stand, and falls upon the side; stretches out the limbs and in a few hours is dead.

The disease is worse on moist rich bottom lands and is rare on dry hills or gravelly soils. To prevent the disease, such soils and localities should be avoided, and the sudden changes from poor to such rich and succulent and abundant pasturage.

The SPECIFIC F F, is the proper remedy, and may be given in doses of five drops to the worst cases every four hours, and to the ailing ones two or three times per day. In the very worst cases the Specific I I may be alternated with the F F, every three hours.

WHEN A NUMBER OF SHEEP or a flock are to receive medicine, the best and most economical, as well as efficient method is as follows: Procure a new or perfectly clean pint bottle and cork, fill it two-thirds full of pure water to which add a *large spoonful or sixty drops* of the proper specific, SHAKE IT THOROUGHLY so as perfectly to medicate the whole mass Of this a dessert spoonful is a dose for a sheep. Paste a proper label on the bottle and use it only for that specific, so as to prevent mistake or confusion.

Red Water.

This disease is mostly known in the West and South-West, and is doubtless the result of exposure a1 unwholesome food It is apt to appear in the late fall, or early winter, when sheep have their feed covered with hoar frost, or are obliged to scrape the snow from it, thus eating large quantities of snow and ice, thus producing a peculiar inflammation of the bowels, or from drinking foul water. Not unfrequently quite a proportion of a flock are suddenly attacked.

The sheep appear dull and stupid, and stagger, carrying their head on one side; the eyes are staring, and they are sometimes blind. The bowels are obstinately costive and death ensues in a few hours. After death the belly of the sheep is found filled with reddish serum.

The SPECIFIC, A A, is the remedy, and may be given a dose of five drops every two, three, or four hours, according to circumstances.

Aphthae or Foot and Mouth Disease.

This disease has prevailed extensively in Europe among flocks and herds, and been at times a most sad visitation. It is more rare in this country, but yet has been known in various sections, and we have no assurance but that under peculiar favoring circumstances it may prevail again, so that its symptoms and treatment should be known.

It is a blood poisoning and is highly contagious under favoring circumstances. It affects sheep, cattle, pigs and rabbits.

The most characteristic appearance is the eruption of watery blisters upon the lips and tongue, and between and around the hoofs. The earlier symptoms are shivering, succeeded by fever, cough, and increased pulse. Then there is failing appetite, tenderness over the loins, slavering from the mouth, and grinding of the jaws. Blisters large and small appear on the mouth and tongue, which break and become raw sores with evident suffering. The feet are swollen and covered with blisters which break, and become sores, causing the animal to walk with difficulty, shake the feet, kick or lie down. If the disease progresses, the sheep rapidly lose condition from inability to eat or move about; all the symptoms increase; the hoofs are sloughed off and even the bones of the feet, leaving only a stump, and ewes in lamb abort.

In favorable cases the symptoms abate gradually, and the disease runs its course in from ten to fifteen days. Animals have it but once.

TREATMENT.—In violent epizootics, it is safest to stamp it out by the slaughter and deep burial of every animal effected, and the removal of those that are well from the affected locality. In any event the affected sheep should at once be separated from the flock, and placed in comfortable quarters where they can be conveniently tended. The specific, I I, may be given in doses of five drops three or four times per day. Prepare in water as noted for AUTHRAX FEVER.

The feet should be washed with soap and water, and then with a weak solution of (Coperas,) sulphate of copper, (1 oz. to a bucket of water), and then dressed with WITCH HAZEL OIL or Carbolic Salve, and bound up to keep out the dirt.

Aphthæ or Thrush.

THRUSH is very frequently connected with foot-rot, either as a symptom or a result. It is manifested by the animal refusing to eat the customary food; dullness; the cud is not chewed; frothy, stringy saliva flows from the mouth, which is found, on examination, covered with small blisters, and the animal grows thin and poor.

TREATMENT.—A few doses of the SPECIFIC for DISTEMPER, C C, given morning and night, will promptly cure. Five drops in water are sufficient for a dose.

Hoove, Fog, Blast, Blown.

This disease is usually occasioned from eating clover, turnips, etc.

SYMPTOMS.—The whole belly is much enlarged the swelling is most manifest at the flanks and on the left side; the swelling is elastic, and gives a hollow sound when struck; the breathing is much impeded and very difficult; the sheep does not eat appears drowsy and sleepy; at last it becomes unconscious, and then dies.

TREATMENT.—The SPECIFIC for WIND BLOWN F F, is perfectly appropriate, and may be repeated every hour until relieved. Five drops may be given as a dose.

Enteritis, Inflammation of the Bowels.

This disease is manifested by the following symptoms: violent and constant pain in the bowels, producing at first uneasiness and then rolling about on the ground; the sheep almost constantly getting up and lying down again; it sometimes lies on its back, the ground is pawed, the belly struck with the hind-feet, etc. These symptoms of pain are attended with confined bowels, quick pulse, cold legs and nose; the belly is tender when pressed upon, and the sheep becomes much reduced in flesh and strength.

TREATMENT.—The SPECIFIC for FEVER, A A, is the appropriate remedy for this disease, and may be given five drops every one, two, or three hours, according to the urgency of the disease.

In cases of extreme distress it may be alternated with the SPECIFIC for COLIC, F F, at intervals of a half-hour or hour, until relieved. But usually the first-named Specific will be quite sufficient.

Dropsy.

Is known as the accumulation of water or servous fluid in the abdomen. It is usually the result of inflammation of the peritoneum or lining membrane of the abdomen. It may be known by the large and pendulous condition of the belly, and by percussing or striking one part of the belly, while the other hand is held against another part, when if water is present the fluctuation is easily perceived. It is caused bi any exposure or food that will produce the origina inflammation.

TREATMENT. " Give five drops of the SPECIFIC, I H, for dropsy three times per day.

Diarrhea.

Purging is most common in spring, and is thei occasioned by fresh grass to which the flock are un accustomed; lambs are subject to a severe and oftei fatal form of this complaint, caused by the irritatioi of grass eaten for the first time. In some instance it may be occasioned by cold or by a peculiar irrita tion of the mother's milk.

SYMPTOMS. " The disease is manifested'by dischargi of various colors, and sometimes very profuse. It i accompanied with loss of appetite and wasting of flesh TREATMENT. " If the discharge is merely the effor of nature to rid the system of some hurtful substance it will require no interference. But if it is excessiv or wasting, three or five drops of the SPECIFIC fo DIARRHEA, F F, given morning and night, will usual ly be sufficient to arrest the disease.

Dysentery, or Flux.

Diarrhea not frequently ends in this form of dis ease; it is also the result of peculiar atmospheri" changes, such as a long term of warm weather abrupt ly terminating in damp cold; or it may be produce" by using fodder spoiled by excessive moisture. SYMPTOMS." At the commencement there are th" usual manifestations of fever, such as dullness, loss o appetite, thirsty dry mouth, increased frequency of pulse, etc. To these are added pain in the belly; frequent attempts to dung, followed by an abundant discharge of slime, mixed with small pieces of hard dung; this slime is exceedingly sticky, and adheres to the parts, often binding the tail over the passage, and quite obstructing it; after the discharge has lasted some time, the animal wastes rapidly until it becomes a skeleton, and the loss of strength is rapid and extreme; the discharge at last becomes black, mixed with blood, and highly offensive, until the sheep dies, worn out by the excessive drain.

TREATMENT.—The animal should be removed from the causes which have induced the disease; the slime must be removed from the tail and thighs with warm water and soap, and sand or fine earth sprinkled on to prevent further adhesion. Give the SPECIFIC for DYSENTERY, F F, five drops three times per day.

Dizziness, Staggers, Sturdy, Turnsick, Gid.

This is a very dangerous and not infrequent disease almost exclusively confined to wool-bearing animals. It is most common in wet, marshy places, and among lambs under a year old. Its immediate cause is the presence of a small worm inclosed in a hydatid or sack of fluid and located either within the substances of the brain, or beneath the bones of the cranium. These hydatids vary in size, number and position, being found on the right or left side, indicated by the animal turning to the right or left, or in the center of the median line, in which case it may turn to either side, or not at all, the animal carrying the head down. When the hydatid occupies the back of the head, the animal holds the head high, and runs straight forward, throwing itself on any object it meets.

SYMPTOMS.—As above indicated, the symptoms consist of various forms of turning, whirling around or standing still, etc. At first, when the hydatids are small there may be but little or nothing to indicate their presence; but as they grow larger, they press upon the bone and even enlarge or remove a great portion of it. One side of the head may be enormously enlarged, or the bone become quite thin so that the situation of the cyst may be thus known, and sometimes a small hole may be discerned. The sacks are more frequently on the left side.

The first effects are dullness, loss of spirits; they chew the cud slowly and carelessly; they keep aloof from the other sheep; they stagger when walking; stand before a pool of water looking into it, and sometimes tumble in and are drowned; sometimes when eating they appear as if frightened, and run over the field as if pursued; the head is held higher or lower or carried on one side; the body in moving inclines to the same side; the eyes have a peculiar bluish color; the sheep appear to wander about, and gradually loose flesh and strength; then they begin to turn round and round to one side; seem quite unconscious of every thing around them; the round and round movements increase until they are almost constant, and the animal at length dies.

TREATMENT.—The old school methods of treatment avail nothing for this disease. Puncturing through the skull into these cysts when their presence is known by the swelling, is sometimes successful of the precise point is known and no other exists. But Homeopathic treatment has been successful. Give the SPECIFIC for FEVER and CONVULSIONS, A A, a dose of two or five drops every night at first, and then at longer intervals, and the symptoms from these parasites sometimes disappear.

In obstinate cases give SPECIFICS, A A and C C, alternately, every four hours may be tried. But the general rule is to slaughter the very decided cases.

APOPLEXY.

23 CHAPTER II.

DISEASES OF THE NERVOUS SYSTEM.

Apoplexy.

In consequence of that phethora which is the re suit of over-feeding in fattening, sheep are quite liabl to apoplexy, and when in this condition they ar driven rapidly some distance in warm weather the are quite liable to a fit of this disease.

SYMPTOMS. " Generally there are some symptom which indicate that an animal is about to have a fi of this very frequent complaint. These are: Duli ness; frequent standing still, or remaining behind th others; the breathing is quickened; it seems sleep and unaware of what is going on around; the eye appear as if they were blind; the pupils are redden ed and nostrils dilated; pulse is quick and hard the membranes of the nose and eyes are red ; ther from standing fixed as it were in one place, it stag gers and falls; then is violently convulsed, and unles relieved death speedily ensues.

TREATMENT " The SPECIFIC for FEVER, A A,: given before the convulsion, a dose of three or fiv drops, will arrest its farther progress.

If the fit has taken place give the medicine at once and repeat the dose again after the animal gets ove it, should it survive the fit.

Encephalitis, Inflammation of the Brain.

This disease may arise from internal causes, but more frequently from sun-stroke, blows upon the head, too plentiful food, etc.

SYMPTOMS.—The animal ceases to eat; hangs its ears and head, which are hot to the touch; walks along staggering, unconscious whither it goes; the eyes are bright and red, and projected from the head; the air it expires is hot; the breathing short, rapid, and accompanied with violent beating of the flanks; it remains lying down, head stretched on the ground, and, as the disease draws to a close, it ends in convulsions.

TREATMENT.—Give the FEVER SPECIFIC, A A, a dose of three or five drops every hour during the height of the disease, and then at longer intervals as the case improves.

PNEUMONIA, INFLAMMATION OF THE LUNGS.

23 CHAPTER III.

DISEASES OF THE ORGANS OF RESPIRATIOH

Pneumonia, Inflammation of the Lungs.

THIS disease may be caused by exposure to col" and wet; too severe weather; sudden changes o weather; cold nights and mornings and hot mid days, are apt to induce it.

SYMPTOMS. " Want of appetite; loss of the cud dull, staring eyes; ears are hung down; the head i held up; the mouth open; breathing quick, labored and difficult, with heaving of the flanks; grating o the teeth; inside of the nose and white of the eye: much reddened; a discharge, at first thin anc watery, afterwards mattery and offensive, flows fron the nostrils; frequent painful cough, attended witl rattling in the throat. These symptoms gradually become more and more severe until the anima dies.

TREATMENT. " The SPECIFIC for FEVER, A. A, wil generally be found sufficient. Give a close of fiv" drops every two hours. Should the disease no yield in a day or two, the SPECIFIC for INFLAMEI LUNGS, E E, in doses of five drops, may be alter nated with the A A, every three hours.

CHAPTER IV.

DISEASES OF THE FEET.

Foot-Rot.

THIS disease is most common in low, marshy places, and results from foreign bodies, such as sand, gravel, sticks, or dirt, getting into the cleft of the foot.

SYMPTOMS.—Lameness, swelling of the pastern, pain, etc.; matter then forms, and unless it is let out, it will spread in all directions under the foot and appear at the coronet; long, narrow ulcers remain, and proud flesh springs up from the diseased places.

TREATMENT.—Examine the foot carefully; remove all dirt or other foreign matter; then foment the foot night and morning with hot water for an hour, and then apply a turnip or bran poultice; the hoof should be pared down, and all the dead parts, or those likely to interfere with the escape of matter, cut away; afterwards apply THE WITCH-HAZEL OIL, on a piece of cloth bandaged to the foot, to keep it in place and prevent dirt or other matter getting into the sore. If the parts are healthy, the ıar and tallow application (equal parts) is very serviceable. The hoof will then begin to grow, during which care must be taken to prevent dirt lodging in the wound and causing fresh irritation. A dose of the SPECIFIC for ULCERS, I I, every morning, and of J J, for condition every night, will aid the process,

FOUNDEE.

24 Founder.

Sheep are occasionally foundered from similar cause which produce it in other animals. It is manifeste" by the following symptoms: It walks slowly; hea" depressed; has no sprightliness; poor appetite, bu great thirst. After a time this slowness of walking becomes a rigidity, so that it requires great effort fo the animal to lie down or get up again. The ap petite diminishes and thirst increases. In the mon advanced stages the eyelids are swollen the eye more or less inflamed, and the feet extremely hot still farther advanced, there is no appetite, feet an burning and hot, the animal is in so much pain fron movement, that it will on]y walk to satisfy its raginj thirst. It drags itself along often on its knees rathe than walk. It moans and groans, there is seven fever, short breathing, and severe beating of tin flanks.

TREATMENT. " The SPECIFIC for FOUNDER, 13 1] will be. sufficient in usual cases. Give three drop three times per day, or morning and night if the cas" is not urgent. If there is heat or fever the SPECIFIC A A, may be given as an intermediate remedy.

CHAPTER V.

GENERAL DISEASES.

Scab or Pock.

This disease, which attacks the same animal but once in life, and by preference the young ones of the flock, is one which sometimes occasions fearful ravages among sheep. It has its regular stages like the small-pox, and may be mild or malignant.

SYMPTOMS.—In the mild form, the animal is for two or three days sad and dejected; then on different parts, more particularly on the inner surface of the fore-feet and around the mouth, small red spots appear, whose center is occupied by a pimple, terminating in a white point. This stage of eruption is attended with feverish shiverings, heat, especially of the ears and nose: redness of the eyes and inner mouth; the animal is melancholy; head down; feet close together; lameness especially of hind parts; no appetite or cud. The greater the number of pustules the worse the disease. The body is hot; breathing short; a clear mucus flows from the mouth; the parts occupied with pimples, especially the head, swell so that the animal can not open its eyes or mouth; the fever continues; the pustules enlarge, and are filled with fluid, first thin, and then becoming thick, yellow, and purulent. On the thirteenth day the pustules begin to dry up, fever abates, pus hardens in the pustules, becomes yellow, then darker, flatten, become scabs, and by degrees fall off, leaving a dry scar behind. The drying stage lasts from five to seven days.

Sometimes this disease assumes a malignant form, in which the pock are very numerous, running together; the symptoms violent, irregular, and the pock soon becomes dark-colored. The pustules run together, forming extensive ulcers beneath the wool, frequently destroying the eyes and entire pieces of the lips and face.

TREATMENT.—During the feverish stage for the first five or six days give the SPECIFIC for FEVER, A A, five drops four times per day. Then give the SPECIFIC for ERUPTIONS, I I, the same dose morning and night, until the animal is well. This SPECIFIC, I I, given to the well sheep will so act as to either prevent their having it at all, or only in a very mild form. The sound and diseased or suspected sheep should be separated, as the disease is very contagious, and easily communicated.

If, however, the disease has appeared in a flock with some severity, inoculation is best, quickest, and safest. This may be done on the forearm or other part with matter from a fresh pock, merely dipping the lancet in it and inserting it just beneath the skin, not so as to cause the blood to flow, or it may wash it out. The advantage is, that all have it lightly, and get over it in three weeks, otherwise the flock may be six months having it; and not one per cent. of inoculated animals will die During the disease they should not be kept too warm or be overfed.

Mange, or Itch

Is quite common in sheep, and assumes a variety of forms. It is especially liable to occur in long-continued rainy, damp weather, and when flocks are long exposed and unsheltered. Small pimples and then vesicles start up, secreting a viscid, glutinous fluid; and in many cases these vesicles run into corroding ulcers, which extend more and more, attended with violent itching and burning.

TREATMENT.—The infected sheep should be separated from the flock, and be placed in a dry, sheltered abode, and given good food and careful attendance, and each day give to each unsound or suspected one, two drops of the ERUPTION SPECIFIC I I. This remedy will generally suffice. If they have been long diseased, it is best to shear them at once. In obstinate cases Dr. Gunther's *Balsamus Terebinthinæ Sulphuratus* has been applied with great success. It may be prepared by any one in the following manner: Dissolve one part, by weight, of sulphur in four parts of linseed oil, by boiling them together over a fire. The result of this will be a black-brown elastic oil, of which mix one part, by weight, with three parts of turpentine, by exposing the two to a gentle heat, and the result is the preparation in question, of which give the diseased animals two drops each day, and they will soon be well.

Rot.

The rot generally appears in the autumn of wet summers, and then continues during winter and spring. The progress of the disease is slow and symptoms as follows:

The animal often remains behind the rest of the flock, and allows itself to be seized without resistance; it walks with a slow gait, with shaking head and depressed ears; the loins yie'd to pressure; the eye is dull and watery; the eyelids are swollen; the lips, gums, and palate have a pale tint; the skin is yellowish, white, and appears puffed, and pits on pressure; the wool changes color, loses its brightness, and easily comes off in large flocks, often taking the skin with it; the dung is soft, urine scanty, of deep red color. Gradually there forms on the upper region of the neck, and on the lower jaw, a soft. indolent tumor, which often appears larger on returning from grazing; sometimes disappears at night, but always returns again by day, and gradually increases in size. By degrees the animal loses appetite, but there is increased thirst; rumination ceases; lachrymation becomes more and more abundant, and the nose is full of viscid mucus. Then the abdomen swells, with dropsy; the animal becomes extremely weak, and wastes daily; remains lying down; pulse is quick and soft; and death takes place with convulsions in the midst of diarrhea and progressive coldness of the extremities. In opening the body fluke-worms are often found in the biliary duct and liver, and a large quantity of serum in the chest and abdomen. The blood is pale and watery.

TREATMENT.—The treatment should, of course, commence by removing all occasional causes of the disease, attending to proper diet, housing, etc. The Specific for ERUPTIONS, I I, will be found perfectly adapted to this cachexy, and may be given in doses of five drops two or three times per day.

PART IV.

DISEASES OF THE HOG

Hog Cholera.

A peculiar and very destructive disease, popularly known as HOG CHOLERA has from time to time appeared in all the great pork raising sections of the United States during the last few years. Its ravages have been so extensive, and the destruction of swine have been so great, that not only have individual veterinary men given much time and attention to its investigation and treatment, but the Legislatures of several States have also designated committees to report upon it with a view to its possible arrest. From these authorized statements and investigations as well as from private information we are enabled to form a very clear idea of the several forms of the disease, and of their proper method of treatment.

The name HOG CHOLERA is not well chosen, as it conveys an erroneous impression of the disease, which has little or nothing of the nature of Cholera about it except, perhaps its epizootic character.

It is essentially an "*Anthrax*" disease, with tendency to rapid decomposition of blood, and disorganization of tissue, and in whatever form it may be manifested this characteristic is apparent. The symptoms are not only not always the same, but are widely different at different seasons, and in different localities and even in different individuals in the same locality; so that we must not always expect to meet with the same train of symptoms.

VARIOUS CAUSES have been mentioned all of which may be summed up in unwholesome conditions of life, in food, drink and surroundings, to which is subsequently added an epizootic influence.

Among the exciting causes are: KEEPING MANY HOGS in CLOSE OF NARROW QUARTERS, some are thus over-laid or over-heated and then suddenly chilled while feeding; the disease rarely or never appears when one or two hogs are kept together; FEEDING SWINE ON THE GROUND, IN THE MUD or in troughs where mud and filth is of necessity eaten with the food; as this condition always causes typhus among people, so it will cause blood poisoning or septic disease among swine. TOO RAPID CHANGE OF FOOD as from poor feed, to good feed, or from good to very good feed, the consequence being that the excretory organs, the liver, kidneys, lungs, glands and skin fail to carry off the proper amount of effete or decomposed matter which hence accumulates, occasioning this poisoning of the blood which constitutes the disease. It is from hence that young shotes are most subject to it, and that it is most fatal among them, and hence most common among swine that have been taken up in the fall, and put suddenly upon very rich heavy feed, before the system has become accustomed to the change. This also explains why it is that the most vigorous and thrifty are attacked, while the poorer ones are generally exempt. OVERHEATING by exposing the herd to very hot sun without shade, or exposing to cold chilly, rainy weather without shelter, or, worse than either, permitting them to overheat or overlay each other in straw stacks or similar close quarters from which reeking with heat, they become chilled by coming out into the bleak wind to feed. Such exposure is almost sure to result in congestion and inflammation of the lungs. KEEPING SWINE TOO DIRTY, the skin being covered with mud, scurf or vermin, thus closing the pores and arresting the natural excretory function. If the function of the skin is thus arrested, the kidneys, lungs, glands, and mucuus and serous membranes, must either perform this extra duty, or disease will result, as it does in "Hog Cholera," and hence these organs are so often found affected in this disease. IMPURE DRINKING WATER into which the drainings of the barn yard run or that which is foul from refuse or stagnant matter, produces typhus in a household and will produce malignant disease in swine.

Lastly, INFECTION FROM BEING WITH SICK OR DEAD SWINE OR EATING OF SUCH. It is even asserted that hogs eating the grass that grows on the ground where the dead of this disease have been buried, will be infected. We must remember that all similar diseases have a tendency to assume an epizootic or prevalent form, and that the more diseased or dead ones there are, the more decided this infectious or epizootic influence becomes. It is always safe, if not imperative, to keep well hogs away from the sick, dying, or dead ones.

SYMPTOMS.—The symptoms are not the same from year to year, nor even during the same epizooty, but are varied by the prevalent genus of the disease and mode of its localization upon the different organs. The more early manifestations are: The eyes look dull and deep set in the head; the hair seems to rise or rough up; the inner corner of the eye is gumed up; the animal seems to be dull and weak; he does not run to his feed, but comes slowly or not at all; he eats as though he had no appetite; holds the nose down close to the ground, or it is drawn to one side; he does not lie down with the other swine, but mopes about by himself, or lies in the sun, instead of the shade; and as the disease progresses he refuses his food altogether. He lies down a good deal, has an unsteady gait, and shows a tendency to bury his head, or even his whole body in the litter. This first or forming stage may continue from a few hours to a day or more, when the condition presents a train of symptoms which are varied according to the localization of the disease.

If it falls upon the brain and spinal cord, with intensity, the pig may give a sudden squeal, and fall down in convulsions and die in a few minutes.

If it falls more upon the throat, windpipe and lungs, then, the ears swell, with swelling along the neck; or the entire neck swells; or a hot painful swelling appears along the throat or windpipe which may even extend down to the fore-legs and along the belly; there is also difficult breathing with much heaving of the flanks which when extreme is called "thumps;" with a wheezy, laborious cough, attended with evident pain, with froth from the mouth and the squeal and grunting is hoarse; a reddish bloody matter flows from the nose, and the dung is dry and pasty; in white hogs, red, (Erysipelas) patches, appear about the neck and breast, with swelling; at first the patches are blood red running together, and later they become blueish, or if the case becomes fatal, a blueish black color: In some cases small blisters or pustules appear along the edges of the lips, mouth and tongue, which are filled with gangrenous corrosive fluid, and later these become of a purple lead or grey color. The hog in attempting to run, sways about or totters and the hind legs give out, so that he sits upon his haunches like a dog, and later the fore legs give out also. If started up, he runs off with a squeal resting on his hind legs with his nose to the ground.

When the morbid process localizes itself more upon the kidney and the lining membrane of the bowels, the *back soon becomes arched*, the animal is drawn up with evident pain, and the belly becomes very tender; there is at first only very scanty wax like or dry dung, or none at all, followed in the more advanced or fatal cases with frequent loose offensive or bloody discharges. Towards the close the heaving of the flanks increases, reddish or frothy matter runs from the mouth and nose, and increasingly offensive discharges from the anus.

DURATION of the DISEASE —Some cases terminate, fatally within two days even in a few hours after the first symptoms were observed, though an earlier stage was doubtless in such cases overlooked. But in general, the average duration of the disease is from five to fifteen days, and some have continued from three to six weeks and have recovered, while others have died from repeated relapses.

TREATMENT.—The best treatment of this disease is to prevent it by proper care and attention to the surroundings of the herd But so soon as a single case has been noticed in a herd the most energetic measures should be taken to prevent the disease extending. To this end the herd should at once be placed in a wide roomy well sheltered lot, or under a shelter if the weather is cold, where they can be kept comfortable and free from severe exposure to cold or wet or great heat. and where they can have good clean litter and a good supply of *pure water.* Their feed should be diminished in quantity, and should be given regularly, and be if possible of a more light and relaxing nature than they have been accustomed to. Care should also be taken that the food is perfectly sweet and sound. The herd should be carefully watched, and any animal that shows the first symptom of the disease *should be carefully separated* from the herd, and given proper food and medicine. Animals properly treated in the earlier stage will, in almost every case, be saved, while those only treated in the more advanced stages will be doubtless less fortunate. The only food allowed, should be good, sweet milk or bran mashes, and to the very sick, only the former. They should be treated gently and kindly, as violence or fright increase the violence of the disease, and easily aggravates a slight attack.

THE MEDICINE FOR THE EARLIER SYMPTOMS, and for the ordinary stage, is the SPECIFIC A A FOR FEVER, INFLAMMATION, &c., of which the full dose for a large hog is ten drops, or half as much for shotes. It may be given three times per day in ordinary cases; or, if the animal is very sick, once in three hours. As preventive or with only slight symptoms, one dose per day is sufficient.

BUT WHERE A NUMBER OF HOGS are to be treated, put one teaspoonful or sixty drops of Specific A A into a new or perfectly clean pint bottle half full of pure water, and after shaking well, give each hog a large spoonful at a dose.

IT IS SUFFICIENT that the medicine be put into the mouth so as to thoroughly wet the tongue. If the pig will drink, give it in a little sweet milk.—(Fluid cannot be turned down a hog's throat without strangling it, as the fluid runs directly into the wind-pipe, if the head is held back.) But as sick swine generally lie quietly on the side, the medicine may be given with the Medicator, or with a spoon be poured quietly within the partly opened mouth.

As a preventive, give the well or slightly ailing ones a dose in a little milk every day, for two or three days.

The SPECIFIC A A, should be continued in the earlier stages and all through the disease, except when there is ERYSIPELAS, or very *rapid sinking*, or *paralysis soon coming* on, when the SPECIFIC I I, should be given in place of the A A, or, the two may be given *in alternation*, at intervals of three hours; that is, first A A, next the I I, then the A A, again and so on—And this is the treatment for the worst or more advanced cases.

When the disease has localized upon the AIR-PASSAGES OR LUNGS as manifested by the frequent cough, heaving of flanks and great difficulty of breathing, the SPECIFIC E E, for Pneumonia, will be better than the SPECIFIC I I, and may be given alternately with the A A, in the same manner as the above.

If the disease falls more upon the BOWELS manifested by bloating, great tenderness, and evident pain, arched back, and frequent offensive or bloody liquid dung,—give the SPECIFIC F F, in alternation, with the SPECIEIC I I, in the more advanced cases, or with the SPECIFIC A A, in the recent ones.

For a paralytic condition, or partial *loss of power in the hind legs*, or for any weakness or want of thrift, remaining after the acute disease has subsided, give the SPECIFIC J J, morning and night, ten drops.

Brain Fever, Frenzy, Inflammation of the Brain.

UNDER this head are included inflammation of the parts within the skull, the brain and membranes investing it. It occurs chiefly in pigs which are full of blood, exceedingly fat, and fed upon the most stimulating food.

SYMPTOMS.—Dullness and depression, less lively than usual, and seldom moving from one place to another. As the disease advances the white of the eye becomes covered with red streaks, the pulse is increased in frequency, the breathing quickened, the strength reduced and the animal runs about from one place to another, evidently unconscious and deprived of the power of seeing. Death soon results, usually with convulsions.

TREATMENT.—Give the SPECIFIC for FEVER, A A, a dose of ten drops, every two or three hours, according to the urgency of the disease.

Strangles or Quinzy,—Angina.

This disease is as dangerous as it is common, and usually comes on very suddenly. It mostly occurs from sudden changes of weather, want of drinking water in times of great heat, or the use of cold or snow-water. It occurs chiefly in hot, imperfectly ventilated, unclean sties. Fat hogs are more subject to it than others, and healthy pigs are said to be affected from diseased ones.

SYMPTOMS.—It begins with swelling of the glands under the throat; in proportion to the extent of this swelling the breathing becomes more difficult and heaving, and the swallowing more painful and obstructed, the pulse is quickened, and a high degree of fever results; the swelling, at first hard and painful when touched, becomes soft, red, and more extended, and mortification is not an unusual result; the mouth is hot, saliva flows from it, and the tongue hangs out red and swollen; the eyes are red, the appetite gone, the teeth are grated, the weakness increases, frequent moans are expressed, and unless relieved, the swelling increases so as to arrest the breathing, and the animal dies.

TREATMENT.—The SPECIFIC for FEVER, A A, will generally be found sufficient, and should be given in doses of ten drops every two hours during the height of the disease, and then at longer intervals as the animal improves.

In extreme or severe cases, or of a very malignant type with strong tendency to mortification or putridity, the SPECIFIC for QUINZY, C C, may be given in alternation with that for FEVER, A A, at the intervals mentioned.

Sniffles, or Common Cold.

Choryza, or Cold in the Head.

This disorder is induced by the same causes as produce it in dogs or sheep—cold, wet weather, changes of weather, exposure, etc..

SYMPTOMS.—Discharge from the nostrils of thin watery fluid, which gradually increases in quantity, and may be mixed with blood, followed by cough, sneezing, difficult swallowing, obstructed breathing, general weakness, loss of appetite, swelling of the nostrils, and contraction of one side of the snout It is liable to lead to disease of the lungs, finally ending in consumption.

TREATMENT —The SPECIFIC for DISTEMPER, C C, will be found efficient. Give a dose of ten drops two or three times per day. In case of much heat or fever a dose or two of the FEVER SPECIFIC, A A, may be interposed or alternated with the former, every three or four hours.

Inflammation of the Lungs, or Rising of the Lights.

This disease may be caused in the hog by the same influences which produces it in other animals, but is very liable to be engendered by the impure air of a sty, when dung and dirty litter are allowed to accumulate and decay; and is more liable to occur in some conditions of the atmosphere than others.

SYMPTOMS.—Shivering of the body, red eyes, hot breath, head stretched forward, quick panting breathing, full, accelerated pulse, frequent or almost constant cough, with discharge of phlegm, sweating in various parts of the body, and tongue thrust from the mouth. All these symptoms increase, and the pig dies.

TREATMENT.—Give the SPECIFIC for FEVER, A A, every three hours a dose of ten drops. Should the disease not yield in the course of forty-eight hours, alternate it with the SPECIFIC for INFLAMED LUNGS, E E, at the same intervals, and continue the two in alternation until cured.

Colic, or Gripes.

This disease is of occasional occurence in hogs, and is of some moment, as it may terminate in inflammation of the bowels, and result fatally.

SYMPTOMS.—Restlessness, rolling on the ground, loud cries of pain, and other symptoms indicative of suffering.

TREATMENT.—Give first the SPECIFIC for COLIC, F F, and if not cured repeat the dose in two hours. If it does not yield, and especially if there is much heat, alternate the SPECIFIC A A, for FEVER, with that for COLIC, F F, dose of ten drops at intervals of an hour or two, until relieved.

Enteritis, or Inflammation of the Bowels.

It may be produced by the same causes which induce it in other animals. It may be known by the following:

SYMPTOMS.—The usual manifestations of pain in the bowels as in colic, except that the pain is here continuous, and is aggravated by rubbing the belly or by moving from one place to another; great pain when the belly is touched, frequent looking towards the belly, and squealing with the pain; other symptoms not differing from that manifested by the dog or sheep.

TREATMENT.—Give the FEVER SPECIFIC, A A, a dose of ten drops every two hours, and continue the treatment until the disease is cured. Sometimes when there is extreme pain a dose or two of the SPECIFIC for COLIC, F F, may be interposed with benefit.

Diarrhœa, or Purging.

The symptoms are so well known as to require no particular description. It may arise from bad food, cold or exposure.

TREATMENT.—The SPECIFIC for DIARRHŒA, F F, will be found quite sufficient Give a dose of ten drops two or three times per day.

Measles

The so-called measles of pigs, or that condition of the skin whence this term is derived, is only the local manifestation of a disease which affects the whole body. The causes are but imperfectly known.

SYMPTOMS.--The earlier symptoms are those of fever, namely, hot dry skin, quick pulse, loss of appetite, hot and dry muzzle, swollen eyelids, red eyes, watery running from the nostrils, short, dry cough, etc. Then there are red risings on the skin in various parts of the body, but especially between the fore legs, and between the hind-legs, and in some cases the skin over these parts sloughs or separates in large pieces, leaving angry sores behind, or it simply peels off without leaving any ulcers.

TREATMENT.—In the earlier stage during the fever, and before the eruption has developed itself, give the SPECIFIC for FEVER, A A, a dose of ten drops every three or four hours, and the disease will be arrested.

After the eruption has come out, alternate the SPECIFIC for FEVER with that for ERUPTIONS, I I, in doses of ten drops, at intervals of four hours, until cured.

Mange.

This disease, consisting of an eruption of pimples and violent itching, is well known, and its successful treatment requires the use of the SPECIFIC for ERUPTIONS, I I, internally, a dose of ten drops morning and night, and the use of the *Arsenical Lotion* (see page 28,) every day.

The skin should be well washed and dried before applying the lotion.

PART V.

DISEASES OF THE DOG.

CHAPTER I.

GENERAL DISEASES.

Distemper.

THIS is one of the most common diseases of the dog, and one that leaves in its train often very serious results. The earlier symptoms are very insidious. There is dullness; loss of appetite, flesh, and strength may be remarked, while purging and vomiting are not uncommon. To this are added a short husky cough, watery eyes, increased redness of the vessels of the eye, sensibility of the eye to light, increased frequency of the pulse. As the disease advances, the animal shivers with the cold, dislikes to be disturbed, seeks warmth, and courts solitude; the bowels are confined; the membrane of the eye covered with a fine net-work of bright red vessels; a thick discharge of matter flows from the eyes; the nostrils are covered with a glassy yellowish fluid; the cough is increased in frequency, and comes on in fits, which terminates in the discharge of a yellow, frothy fluid from the stomach; the skin is hot.

A later stage is marked by an increase of all the foregoing symptoms. The body wastes, the shivering is constant, the eyes are filled with a thick matter, which glues the eyelids together in the morning; tenacious matter clogs the nostrils and obstructs the breathing. This causes much uneasiness and frequent but unsuccessful attempts to overcome the cause of annoyance. The discharge from the nostrils becomes bloody and offensive; the breath is fetid; the lips are covered with ulcers; short cries express pain; and the animal, becoming weaker and worse in every respect, at last dies, a severe diarrhœa being the usual harbinger of that end.

Distemper frequently results in chorea, or St. Vitus' dance, paralysis, disease of the brain, ulcers on the eyes and opacity, inflammation of the lungs, or in numerous other ailments.

Treatment.—The earlier stages, before the discharge is established, are best controlled by the Specific for Fever A A, of which give a dose of three or five drops, according to the size of the dog, morning, noon and night.

After the catarrhal stage has come on, give three or five drops of the Specific for Distemper, C C, four times per day. This will in general carry the animal safely and speedily through this ordeal. Should other diseases declare themselves they should be treated accordingly.

Should a general or partial paralysis occur, or inability to use one or several limbs, the Specific, J J, should be given, three or five drops, three times per day until recovered. See Paralysis.

Inflammation of the Bladder, Cystitis.

This disease, which is a very dangerous and painful one, may be caused by stones in the bladder, injuries, fall upon the bladder when it is full of water, or similar accidents.

SYMPTOMS.—Hot, dry skin, pain in the back and flanks, thirst, no appetite, restlessness and signs of pain, frequent attempts to pass water, in which either one or only a few drops are passed at a time; the water may be clear, or thick and mixed with blood.

TREATMENT.—Give first two or three doses of the SPECIFIC for FEVER, A A, at intervals of two hours, then give the SPECIFIC for INFLAMED KIDNEYS and BLADDER, H H, a dose of three or five drops, according to the size of the dog, until entirely relieved, at intervals of two or three hours.

Gonorrhea, Gleet.

This disease, which is essentially an inflammation of the urethra, generally arises from taking the disease by connection with other animals that has it, or from repeated acts of sexual connection, which induces irritation, followed by a gleety discharge; or it may arise in a modified form from uncleanliness.

SYMPTOMS.—Discharge from the internal surface of the sheath and urethra, or canal through which the water flows, consisting of matter having a yellowish or greenish color, glueing together the parts or hair about them; the surface looks red and angry, and is attended with swelling and pain; there is frequent desire to pass water; sometimes the swelling and pain are but slight.

TREATMENT.—Give the SPECIFIC for INFLAMED URETHRA, H H, a dose of three or five drops, according to the size of the dog, four times per day.

In the old cases a dose of the SPECIFIC for DISTEMPER, given nightly, will be of decided benefit.

Inflammation of the Eye, Ophthalmia.

It may arise from a variety of causes, such as congestion of the brain; exposure to heat and cold; over-exertion; blows or other injuries; over-salted food, etc.

SYMPTOMS.—The white of the eye is covered with red streaks; the clear portion in front (pupil) is dim; water runs down the face; the light can not be endured, and the eyelid is closed. An ulcer may appear afterwards in the front of the eye, and it may go on until it penetrates through the outer coating of the eye (cornea), and the fluids of the eye thus escape. In some cases proud flesh springs up from these ulcers.

TREATMENT.—The SPECIFIC A A, for INFLAMMATION, should be given, a dose of two drops only, two or three times per day. This in general will be sufficient for all forms of Ophthalmia; but if the case is of some standing, or if ulcers or degenerations have taken place, two drops of the SPECIFIC for ULCERS, I I, may be given every night, and that for INFLAMMATIONS in the morning, with the best possible results.

A wash of HAMAMELIS diluted one half with soft water, will promptly relieve, and also accelerate the cure.

Canker in the Ear.

This disease consists of an inflammation of the internal ear, followed by ulceration and the formation of matter. It is usually the consequence of some injury, but may also result from excess of food and want of exercise, or from frequent and sudden exposure, as in case of dogs taught to go in the water, among whom it is quite common; fat dogs are more subject to it than others.

SYMPTOMS.—The dog manifests pain by shaking his head, scratching his ears, or whining. The internal ear looks red, afterwards may ulcerate; a disoharge occurs, and a blackish fluid will be found at the bottom of the ear, sometimes in considerable quantity; there is high fever, which, with the continuance of the discharge, may wear out the dog.

TREATMENT.—Wash the ear frequently with warm water, to carefully remove the discharge; afterwards apply some diluted MARVEL.

Give the SPECIFIC for FEVER A A, three or four drops alternately with that for ULCERATIONS, I I. The same does four times per day; it may be successful.

Inflammation of the Ear.

This sometimes occurs from insects having made their way into the ear, sometimes from Rheumatism. The dog complains, shakes his head, scratches his ear, howls, is restless and unquiet, and seeks for aid.

TREATMENT.—The ear should be carefully examined in the light of the sun, and if insects are discovered they should be removed, or destroyed by means of oil applied to the place, and afterwards washed out with warm water.

Give also the SPECIFIC for FEVER, A A, five, drops two or three times per day, to allay the irritation.

Chest-Founder Kennel Lameness.

This is a rheumatic complaint not unfrequent among dogs, and is usually the result of exposure to cold and damp, especially when the animal is warm, or has been over-heated.

SYMPTOMS.—The animal is lame and stiff especially in the fore-legs ; the pain may be so severe that he can not move them, There is pain when the shoulders and sides are pressed upon. There is fever, hot skin, quick pulse, rapid breathing, and loss of appetite.

TREATMENT.—The SPECIFIC for FEVER, A A, should be given at first, a dose of three or five drops, four times per day, while the fever and heat are violent, after which the SPECIFIC for FOUNDER, B B, may be alternated with it at the same intervals until the animal is cured.

Fractures.

Simple fractures of the leg are very readily cured in young and vigorous dogs It may be readily known by the distortion of the limb, by the ends of the bone grating upon each other, lameness, etc.

TREATMENT is very simple. Extend the limb and put the bones in place, and apply splints with a firm bandage, wetting the limb with the MARVEL. Examine them from time to time to see that they are kept in place. After three or four weeks they may be removed, and the animal trusted to use its limbs. Give the SPECIFIC for Injuries, B B, night and morning for a few days; three or five drops according to the size of the animal.

Sore Feet.

These may be occasioned by injuries, long traveling over rough or frozen ground, or in very dry weather.

SYMPTOMS.—The foot is swelled, and small hard, painful lumps are felt in it; there is much pain, and the animal cannot bear its weight upon them. The skin becomes red, and the nails fall off. There is usually considerable fever and no desire to eat.

TREATMENT.—Bathe the feet three or four times per day in the MARVEL, or in Arnica, (See page 27,) and give morning and night a dose of three or five drops of the FEVER SPECIFIC, A A.

If matter forms, a poultice may be applied, and the abscess afterwards opened.

CHAPTER II.

DISEASES OF THE AIR-PASSAGES.

Ozena, or Running from the Nose.

THIS disease is very common in old dogs, and especially in pugs. It is known by a constant discharge from the nostrils, which is bad-smelling, like matter, attended with cough, snorting, attempts to sneeze, obstructed nostrils, and difficulty of breathing. If neglected it may injure or even destroy the sense of smell.

TREATMENT.—The SPECIFIC for DISTEMPER, NASAL DISCHARGES, C C. is perfectly appropriate for such cases. Give a dose of two or five drops, according to the size of the dog, two or three times per day.

Catarrh or Cold, Bronchitis.

It occurs most commonly in the variable weather of winter, and early spring, and is induced from causes similar to those which induce it in the human system.

SYMPTOMS.—There is cough; running from the eyes, which become red; then watery discharge from one or both nostrils; dullness and sleepiness; poor appetite; sneezing; quick, heavy breathing; weakness and wasting.

If the disease is not checked, Bronchitis, or cold in the chest comes on, known by a mattery discharge from the nose, which may be stuffed up, with difficulty of breathing; the breathing is quick, attended with rattling in the windpipe; the cough becomes more frequent and severe

TREATMENT.—Give three or five drops of the SPECIFIC for FEVER, A A, three or four times per day, to allay the heat and feverish excitement, after which a few doses of the SPECIFIC for COUGHS AND COLDS, E E, will complete the cure.

Inflammation of the Chest, Pneumonia or Pleurisy.

Inflammation of the chest usually involves both the pleura or lining membrane of the chest, and the substance of the lungs, so that they may be advantageously treated. It is usually the result of cold and exposure after being heated; it may also be produced by wounds.

SYMPTOMS.—Shivering chill, followed by heat and thirst; the sides are painful when pressed upon; stitches are observed; the dog sits upon his haunches, with the fore-legs separated from each other, and the head held forward; the breath hot; cough short and painful; breathing frequent, labored and heaving; pulse full and quick; tongue hangs out of the mouth; eyes thrust forward and red; finally drowsiness and death. Sometimes the effusion of water in the chest is very abundant, when the legs swell, and breathing becomes difficult, labored and suffocating.

TREATMENT.—Give first three or five drops, according to the size of the dog, of the SPECIFIC for FEVER A A, and repeat the dose every two hours for the first twenty-four hours.

Then alternate the SPECIFIC for INFLAMED LUNGS, E E, with that for Fever at intervals of two or three hours, until the animal is cured.

CHAPTER III.

DISEASES OF THE DIGESTIVE ORGANS

Salivation.

MERCURY, in its various forms, is sometimes given to dogs by ignorant persons, or by chemists and dog-fanciers, for some real or supposed disease; or it is applied to them externally as an ointment for mange, in either case resulting in salivation, with the following

SYMPTOMS.—Loss of appetite; sore, swollen gums, which are blueish, easily bleed, and generally ulcerate; loosened teeth, which may even fall out; constant dribbling of slaver from the mouth; offensive breath; swelled glands; extreme weakness; hair falls off, and frequently purging, attended with straining.

TREATMENT.—Give the SPECIFIC for FEVER, A A, a dose each morning and noon, and a teaspoonful of THE MARVEL at night, especially if there is ulceration of the mouth or throat. If not improved after three or four days substitute SPECIFIC I I, three or five drops, morning and night, which continue until cured.

Diseases of the Teeth.

The teeth are more frequently affected in the dog than in other domestic animals. This may be the result of a variety of causes, among which are the following: Eating or gnawing bones by means of which the teeth may be broken or ground down to the quick; healthy, well-fed dogs only pick their bones; rich, sweetened food, which has an injurious effect upon the teeth; mercury, frequently given to dogs, which produces salivation, loosening, and eventually falling out of the teeth. Teaching dogs to carry or chase hard substances, stones, etc., frequently results in diseased teeth, as they are thus rubbed down to the gum, and the stump produces much mischief.

SYMPTOMS.—If the dog has a bad breath, seems to be in pain when he eats, does not thrive, or manifest his usual spirit, the mouth should be examined. One or more teeth will be found worn down to the gum; the fang produces irritation, and may result in an abscess; the sides of the mouth are raw and ulcerated, and slaver dribbles from it.

TREATMENT.—Extraction is the sole remedy for loose, irregular, or decayed teeth.

Colic.

Colic is not unfrequent in the dog. It is often connected with constipation, and may result from bad food, sudden change of food, exposure to cold or from worms. It is common in puppies.

SYMPTOMS.—The dog has sudden pain in the bowels; it comes on in fits, is worse at one time than another. The dog is restless, frequently changing his position; he extends himself and then draws himself in, turns his head towards his sides, throws himself down, rolls about, moans or whines, when the pain is severe, with a short, rough voice.

TREATMENT.—The SPECIFIC for COLIC, F F, should be given, a dose from three to five drops, according to the size of the dog, and repeated every half-hour or hour as the urgency of the case demands.

Should it not promptly relieve, the SPECIFIC for FEVER, A A, or that for CONSTIPATION, J J, may be given alternately with that for COLIC.

Constipation, or Bound Bowels.

Constipation is more frequently observed than diarrhea in a dog. It may be the result of a want of proper exercise, improper food, or some disorder of the liver or other part of the digestive system. It is manifested by frequent unavailing efforts to evacuate, attended with groaning, trembling, or other manifestations of pain. It may result in mange or even inflammation unless relieved.

TREATMENT—Give the SPECIFIC for CONSTIPATION, J J, three to five drops, according to the size of the animal, three times per day.

Should this course not relieve, an injection of warm soap and water should be given, and repeated if necessary until the result is accomplished.

Diarrhea.

Excess of food, bad food, exposure to cold and wet, as well as a bilious condition, may induce diarrhea in the dog. If slight it will cure itself. It usually manifests itself by sickness, vomiting, thirst, discharges more frequent and thinner than usual. If it continues, the animal becomes thin, weak, does not eat his food and his breath becomes offensive.

TREATMENT. — The SPECIFIC for DIARRHEA, F F, will be found effectual. Give three or four drops, according to the size of the dog three times per day.

Dysentery.

It is not unfrequently a termination of diarrhea, or it may be produced by similar causes.

SYMPTOMS.—Thirst, heat, purging of fluid mixed with small pieces of dung, attended with severe straining and pain; often the discharges are of mucus mixed with blood. There is loss of strength and appetite, with rapid wasting.

TREATMENT.—Give the SPECIFIC for DYSENTERY, F F, two to five drops every one, two or three hours, according to the urgency of the case.

Inflammation of the Bowels.

Neglected or improperly treated colic, exposure to cold and damp after fatigue, or stones in the bowels may produce this disease.

SYMPTOMS.—The belly is hot, painful and contracted; it is very painful on contact or pressure; the dog moves slowly with fear and trembling; he cries or howls with pain; does not eat, but is very thirsty; looks around at his belly; his bowels are very confined; dung is hard and in small pieces; cold legs; the tail is kept down close between the legs.

TREATMENT.—Give the SPECIFIC for FEVER and INFLAMMATION, A A, three or five drops, according to the size of the dog, and repeat it every hour or two hours, according to the urgency of the case. Sometimes a dose of the SPECIFIC for COLIC, F F, may be interposed, or given alternately with that for FEVER, with advantage.

Inflammation of the Liver, Jaundice.

This disease is occasionally found in dogs, more particularly in fat ones. It may be the result of excess of food and deficient exercise, or exposure to cold or moisture.

SYMPTOMS.—The dog is dull, sleepy, shrinks from notice, and becomes thin; eats little and is thirsty. The skin, gums, lips, and parts of the skin not covered with hair are yellow; the urine is yellowish and dung dark-colored, hence the name *Jaundice* or yellows. He is sometimes hot, at others cold; he vomits a yellow fluid, which may afterwards become greenish, and have streaks of blood in it. These symptoms all increase until the dog becomes thin as a skeleton, and at last dies quite worn out.

TREATMENT.—Give the SPECIFIC for FEVER, A A, alternately with that for JAUNDICE, J J, a dose of three to five drops, according to the size of the dog, every three or four hours, as the urgency of the case may demand.

Old cases of liver complaint simply require a dose of the SPECIFIC for JAUNDICE, J J, morning and night.

Worms.

No animal is so subject or so frequently tormented by worms as the dog. This is doubtless owing to his highly artificial life and the great variety of food given him. There are three varieties: The first is red, resembling the earth-worm, and is common in puppies; the second is the *tenia* or tape-worm, which is sometimes of great length, flat, in joints, and occupies the small intestines; the third is the *ascarides* or pin-worm, half an inch to an inch in length, thread-like, pointed, and housing in the lower part of the bowels.

SYMPTOMS.—All worm symptoms are questionable except finding them in the discharges. Their existence may be inferred if the dog has a short, dry cough, bad breath, greedy appetite, rough coat, bound bowels or purging, turns of griping, wasting, or fits.

TREATMENT.—Give the SPECIFIC for WORMS, D D, two to five drops, according to the size of the dog, two or three times per day. Its continuance will not fail to eradicate them from the system.

CHAPTER IV.

DISEASES OF THE NERVOUS SYSTEM.

Epilepsy, or Fits.

The dog is occasionally subject to true epilepsy, and not unfrequently to fits or convulsions arising from transient causes; such as teething in puppies, worms, want of exercise, and then too violent exercise. They are liable also to come on during distemper or after it, or from disease of the brain. Small pet dogs are more subject to fits than others, as their nervous system is more excitable and their lives more artificial.

SYMPTOMS.—The fit generally comes on suddenly, the animal staggers, falls down, remains lying for an instant, and then is violently convulsed; the legs become stiff, the face distorted, the eyes roll about, the tongue is thrust out, the jaws nearly closed or firmly clenched. The convulsion becomes gradually less, and after some twitches they cease, and the animal in a short time appears well again.

In true epilepsy the fits recur again at diminishing intervals, and excitements may easily reproduce them.

TREATMENT.—Give, on an attack from whatever cause, from two to five drops, according to the size of the animal, of the SPECIFIC for CONVULSIONS, A A, and repeat it once after the paroxysm is over. This will be sufficient for fits arising from any transient cause; but if the dog is subject to them he must have the SPECIFIC J J for PARALYSIS, alternately with that for CONVULSIONS, A A, a dose every day or two, and continued for some time to effect a radical cure.

Chorea, St. Vitus' Dance.

This is a frequent result of severe distemper, especially in the case of young dogs, and it may also arise from worms or some disorder of the stomach.

SYMPTOMS.—The disease manifests itself by twitches, or involuntary jerks of various parts, as the leg, shoulder, face, neck, or even eyelids. Sometimes it is confined to a single limb or two, or the whole body may be affected The animal has no control over them, and they are manifested even during sleep. He wastes, eats, and sleeps badly and may become palsied; at last he becomes incapable of any service, staggers, has convulsions, and is at last worn out.

TREATMENT.—Give the SPECIFIC for CONVULSIONS, A A, each morning, and that for PARALYSIS, J J, each night, two to five drops, according to the size of the animal, and follow the treatment perseveringly.

Palsy, Paralysis.

This is not an unfrequent affection in the dog, especially those that are well fed, as pet dogs. It arises from disease of the brain or spinal cord, and is sometimes also the result of disease of the bowels or stomach.

SYMPTOMS.—It may occur in one side or part of the animal, and is most frequent in the hind-legs, which appear as if the animal had no power over them; he staggers, falls, or lies on the ground, dragging his hind-legs after him, unable to stand upon them.

TREATMENT.—Give the SPECIFIC for PARALYSIS, J J, two to five drops, according to the size of the dog, three times per day.

In case it comes on suddenly in well fed dogs, from an over-feed or gorging the animal, give a spoonful of castor oil and an injection of warm soap and water, followed with the prescription above.

Rabies, Canine Madness.

Much has been said upon the subject of *Rabies*, or *Canine Madness*, and from the general horror in which the disease is justly held, some consideration of it is proper, even if we do not possess the means of cure. The causes of the disease are involved in obscurity, yet it may be spontaneous or communicative. The former has been attributed to want of care, deficient water in hot weather, intense heat or cold, an inability to satisfy the venereal appetite If communicated, it is from the saliva of the affected dog, in which case the disease seldom breaks out before the ninth day, often later. Two principal forms of this disease have been distinguished: rabies proper, and dumb madness.

SYMPTOMS of Rabies proper:—First change noticed is in the dog's gait in walking, either more lively and irritable than usual, or more dull and sad; peculiar restlessness; does not remain in one place; often quits his home and roams to a distance; he recognizes and obeys his master at the commencement, and even through the entire disease, generally no appetite from the commencement; some will take soup, but never solid food; they often, however, devour strange things, as wood, leather, straw, or even filth; they drink in all stages of the disease as long as they can swallow; there is always a peculiar change of voice, more shrill or more grave, always slightly hoarse and disagreeable; the bark is peculiar, not in distinct emisions, as in health, but an emission of voice ending in a howl; the desire to bite is not constant, but comes occasionally in fits, and varying degrees; during the fits he bites every thing, cats, other dogs, human beings, even his own master, or inanimate objects, and frequently snaps at the air. At first he is but little changed in appearance; but soon the eyes become red; they open and shut alternately; later, they are dull, as if covered with dust; sometimes the skin wrinkles on the forehead, or the head swells; rapid emaciation; he becomes finally very weak, and drags his hind-quarters; while at first he is strong, carries his tail as usual, and differs not in gait from a healthy dog.

The other form of madness is manifested by loss of appetite, drink, voice, and manifestation of the passion for biting as in the first instance, modified thus: The lower jaw droops, apparently paralyzed from the commencement; he can not swallow any liquid; saliva constantly flows from his mouth; the tongue often hangs from between the teeth; he bites less than in the first form; still, as there are times when irritated that he may close his mouth, the danger from biting is the same.

There are some popular errors which are corrected by the following statements, thus: Dogs may become mad at any season of the year. Female and altered dogs may become mad by communication, though the disease originates probably with entire animals. Mad dogs drink in all stages of the disease, if the soreness of the throat, or paralysis of the jaws, or flow of saliva, does not prevent them; they have even been known to swim in water. Mad dogs do not always carry the tail between the legs, but otherwise, during the commencement of the disease; it is, however, common in many other diseases, and in all dogs when pursued or frightened. Mad dogs do not always run in a straight line, unless pursued; they change their direction like other dogs, and run to objects which attract them. Other dogs do not avoid them, but if a stranger, it will be attacked by well dogs Sound animals have no repugnance to the saliva of a mad dog, but will even eat meat which is covered with it.

TREATMENT.—All the means hitherto discovered to arrest the disease have proved unreliable BELLADONNA and the SPECIFIC for CONVULSIONS may do something, and had best be administered in all doubtful cases; but if an animal is indisputably rabid it should be killed at once. The excision of the gland or ligament under the tongue is only mutilating the animal to no purpose.

If a dog is suspected or has been bitten, or exposed to contagion, give him the SPECIFIC for CONVULSIONS, A A, three or four drops, according to his size, three times per day, and inject a dose of the same medicine into the wound at the same time. Only a small proportion of the animals or persons bitten by animals supposed to be rabid ever become mad.

CHAPTER V.

DISEASES OF THE SKIN.

Small Pox.

THIS disease is most common in puppies before the sixth month, and is most severe in hot weather, or when dogs are kept very warm. A very cold atmosphere prevents its coming to the surface, in which case the animal is likely to die from congestion. It is strictly contagious, and is communicated from one dog to another very rapidly.

SYMPTOMS.—First there is a severe fever and perceptible oppression of the breath, after which the skin on the belly, groins, and between the forelegs, becomes red, and then covered with small, round pimples, distinct or clustered in groups. The pimples gradually increase until the fifth day, when the top of each contains a clear fluid, which by degrees becomes yellow, the tops of the pustule then become flat, and by degrees hollowed, and either break and discharge their contents, or dry and form scabs. These by degrees fall or are rubbed off, leaving the skin covered with brown spots or small sores, which remain, removing the hair and leaving the skin bare. When the pustules break, the breath and all the excretions have a bad smell, and inflammation of the lungs is apt to set in.

TREATMENT.—Keep the dog cool during the feverish stage in a well-aired room, and not by the fire; thus the pock will be much less; and give every three hours from two to five drops of the SPECIFIC for FEVER, A A., according to the size of the dog.

After the feverish symptoms have abated, and the pock have come out, give from two to five drops, according to the size of the animal, of the SPECIFIC for ERUPTIONS, I I, three or four times per day, until the cure is complete.

Vermin, Lice.

Lice often cover the body of the dog, especially crowding upon his head, around the eyes and lips. There need be no fear of their presence, as they will not live upon the human being.

TREATMENT.—Mayhew advises to place the dog in a room where grease is not of much moment, and to completely saturate him with castor oil, rubbing it well into the hair on every part. In this state he should be allowed to remain twelve hours, after which the oil should be removed with the yoke of eggs and water. A pint of oil will be required for a moderate-sized dog with long hair, and four times as much for a large Newfoundland dog.

Mange.

Mange is quite common in dogs, especially those that are over-fed, indolent, and have not particular attention paid them. It is induced by confinement in a close or dirty kennel, certain kinds of food, indolence, too much food and too little exercise, starvation; or it may be taken by a healthy dog from a mangy one, or transmitted from a mother to her puppies.

SYMPTOMS.—It may be either dry or moist; the skin is itchy; the dog always rubbing himself, so that the skin is bare and red in different places; along the back small-reddish pimples arise, which are afterwards covered with branny scales. In the moist form there is swelling, redness of the skin, and then secretion of thick puriform mucus, finally formation of matter and thick scabs. The dog becomes thin, low-spirited, and finally dies, unless relieved.

TREATMENT.—Give the SPECIFIC for MANGE, I I, three or five drops, according to the size of the dog, night and morning.

Apply the Arsenical Lotion (See page 28) thoroughly night and morning.

DISEASES OF POULTRY

Doses and Methods of Preparing the Specifics for Use.

ONE DROP or PART of a DROP is quite sufficient as a dose for an ordinary fowl. One drop of any specific put into a teaspoonful of water, or milk, and this put into a teacup so as to *be thoroughly mixed*, is a sufficient dose for FIVE FOWLS of full size or ten chickens.

WHERE a FLOCK or several fowls are to be treated, drop ten drops of the proper specific into a cup, to which add ten teaspoonsful of water, milk, or curdled milk, and after *stirring it thoroughly* with a perfectly clean spoon, mix this with the meal, grain, or bread, or whatever food is given them. If the quantity of fluid should not be sufficient to properly moisten the food, more can be added without detriment, provided the mass be *thoroughly stirred and mixed* before wetting the food. This would be enough for fifty fowls. Some will get more and some less, of course; but each will probably get enough to answer a curative purpose, and none will get so much as to be injurious.

If a bird is so ill as not to eat or drink, and the Specific must be given by hand, the mouth may be gently opened and two or three drops of the mixture made in the proportion of one drop of the Specific to a *teaspoonful* of water may be turned down, or the fluid may be turned on soft food and thus given at the intervals mentioned under each separate disease.

Bread soaked in milk or water, cooked cracked wheat, or curdled milk, is in general the best food for sick or ailing fowls.

DISEASES OF FOWLS.

Cold and Cankered Mouth and Throat.

The more common results of a cold in fowls is a peculiar condition of the head and eyes, which at first appear red and irritated about the eyes and mouth, which by degrees become swelled, and then the nose, mouth and throat become ulcerated or filled up with canker. Sometimes the eyes seem affected with inflammation and partial blindness and there is difficult breathing or rattling of mucus or canker in the throat. At times the entire head is swelled, and the nose and throat are filled with thick cheesy mucus or canker, or pustules appear on the sides of the head, the wattles and ear lobes. As the pustules break or fall off, scales form on the surface. In its more advanced stages the disease is often termed "ROUP."

The SPECIFIC, A A, is required at first in the more inflammatory stages. But after the CANKER has fully formed the SPECIFIC, C C, is the proper remedy. The medicine should be given four times per day, or every say four hours, or for slight attacks morning and night. A wash of salt and vinegar applied to the ulcerated or cankered surface with a suitable swab, is sometimes recommended. But if the disease is cured by the proper specific the ulcer and canker will disappear.

Apoplexy and Paralysis.

May arise as a result of overfeeding or too rapid change of condition. An unsteady gait and drooping wing is the warning. If it progresses there may be entire loss of power or unconsciousness. A dose of SPECIFIC, A A, will afford prompt relief.

Black Rot

is known by a blackening of the comb and swelling of the feet and legs. The SPECIFIC, C C, given three times per day is the proper remedy, and given early may avert the disease.

Bronchitis

Is known by the frequent coughing, and if observed, a more frequent respiration than in health, and generally a well marked rattling in the throat may be noticed. In the more advanced stage there is discharge as in catarrh, or a slight discharge as it gets well.

The SPECIFIC A.A. will promptly cure. Give two or three times per day.

Bumble Foot

Occurs mostly in the large breeds of fowls, and is supposed to be caused by bruising the foot when alighting on a hard surface, or in resting on a small or uneven perch. There is a swelling or corn in the bottom of the foot which softens, becomes ulcerated, forming a putrid surface or sore. Remove the putrid or decayed matter carefully, and dip the foot in a solution of (blue vitriol) sulphate of copper, made by dissolving one-fourth ounce of blue vitriol in a quart of water; this may be repeated two or three times, and give also internally the SPECIFIC, J J, or if the foot is hot and swelled and not yet maturated, the SPECIFIC, A A, may dissipate the swelling without its maturating The bird should be kept on the straw and not suffered to rest on the perch.

Canker or Ulceration.

This disease differs from roup in there being no discharge from the nostril. Ulcerations are found in the mouth involving the tongue and throat. The fowls should have only soft feed, and be kept in warm, dry, clean quarters, and should have the SPECIFIC, C C, three times per day.

Cholera

Usually makes its appearance, as a diarrhea, with frequent greenish droppings, and violent thirst, and extreme weakness and rapid failing of strength; the birds staggering or falling about, and often attacks of cramps. There is generally also an anxious look in the face. The disease is sometimes rapidly fatal death occurring in one or two days.

It is generally admitted to be caused by confining too many birds in close limited quarters, insufficient shade, stale, unhealthy drinking water, exposure to the hot sun, feeding on grass-runs covered with droppings, and the want also of a regular supply of fresh green food. The disease rarely or never occurs where fowls have a liberal range, clean runs, good water, and green food daily.

TREATMENT.—The flock should at once be removed from their unhealthy surroundings and be given a clear, ample range, and should only be allowed a wholesome food of boiled milk thickened with flour, or soft bread soaked in boiled milk, or other suitable food, and should have the SPECIFIC, F F, every three hours in urgent cases, or three times per day to those who are yet able to eat.

Catarrh.

A catarrh is usually the result of a common cold, and is known by the discharge of mucus from the nose. If neglected, it may end in "ROUP." The bird should be removed to a warm, comfortable place, and given the SPECIFIC C.C. three times per day, with bread soaked in milk as food.

Consumption

is sometimes observed in fowls, manifested by cough, wasting of flesh, and great weakness, notwithstanding good feed. It may arise from breeding too much "in and in," but most commonly results from a neglected cold, and bad surroundings. The proper treatment is give the bird good care and feed and the use of SPECIFIC E E, three times per day.

Cramp.

Chickens are sometimes subject to this disease, especially in damp, cold weather. The toes are first seen to be bent under, and by degrees they walk on he knuckles or outside of the foot, and the birds ften squat on the hock. If it is the result of a cold and the chickens are feverish, as is generally the case, remove them to a comfortable place and give them the SPECIFIC, A A, three times per day. If it fails after a day or two try the SPECIFIC J J. If the toes are badly cramped they may be washed in warm water and gently opened and kneaded by the fingers and afterwards be wiped dry.

Crop Bound.

We should distinguish whether the over-distention of the crop is from excessive drinking, and caused by a peculiar feverish condition, or from the bird gorging itself with grain, tough meat or bone too large to be digested. When the crop is so distended with hard food or other substance, the outlet is narrowed or entirely closed so that mechanical manipulation may be necessary to cause its passage. While in the case of distention by fluid the distention will disappear and the unnatural craving for drink will yield to a few doses of the SPECIFIC A A, given at intervals of a few hours.

Where the crop is distended with hard food, and is not passing off and help is required, pour some milk warm water down the throat, and then holding the head downward quietly manipulate or knead the distended crop with the hand so as to soften the mass. After the mass has thus been carefully softened pour down a large teaspoonful of castor or sweet oil, and the mass will be gradually worked off. Food should not be allowed for some time. Give also the SPECIFIC, J J, for indigestion two or three times a day, which may be continued to entire recovery. In many cases the use of the SPECIFIC J J, will be successful without the use of any other means.

Debility Drooping

Occasionally, without apparent cause, except from long continued fright, long journeys, exhibition, or other unnatural condition, the bird droops, mopes about, becomes debilitated, and may die without apparent disease Give first the SPECIFIC, A A, for fright or excitement morning and night for three or four days, and then the SPECIFIC, J J, for indigestion and debility for some days in the same manner, and the two may be thus used alternately if needful.

Diarrhea and Dysentery (Scouring)

Is not uncommon among fowls, caused usually by improper food or sudden changes of weather or severe exposure. In diarrhea the droppings are only too frequent, watery, scalding or excessive, with consequent drooping and wasting of flesh; while, if this condition is unchecked, the discharges become bloody, or mingled with blood and mucus, forming a real *dysentery*. This latter form of the disease is said to be contagious and requires that the diseased birds should be separated from the flock and the dead ones buried deeply far away from the yards or pens of the flock. The treatment is the same, the SPECIFIC F F, should be given three or four times per day. The food should be boiled milk thickened with flour, and well cooked in the worst cases, or good bread softened in scalded milk. Of course the birds should have a clean, dry, and well littered and sheltered place

Egg Bound.

Sometimes hens are unable to drop the egg from its unusual size. This is usually manifested by the hens coming off the nest and moping around with the wings down and in evident distress. A large spoonful of castor or olive oil often relieves, to which should be added a dose of SPECIFIC G G. Should this fail after an hour, bathe the vent with warm water, and then with a feather dipped in oil lubricate or freely oil the passage or viaduct, taking care not to break the egg. Should the egg passage be ruptured or protruded, the SPECIFIC I I, may be given one or two doses to promote the healing.

Eruptions, or Scaly Legs.

Fowls are at times subject to eruptions, sometimes like a whitish bran-like scurf over the head and body; or a rough scurf on the legs and toes like scales. These eruptions are usually the result of confinement in insufficient, damp, wet or muddy runs, and they may in extreme cases be infectious, or be communicated from one fowl to another. The internal use of SPECIFIC I I, given morning and night will insure a cure, if the birds are given good wholesome food, and have a clean run of grass and suitable shelter. If the eruptions are unsightly a little plain sweet oil applied with a feather will effect their removal, but the cure must be by the use of the specific given in the feed.

Feather Eating.

This unnatural appetite, mostly observed in the hen, is the expression of some chemical want in the system, which, not satisfied in the food or drink of the fowl, manifests itself in picking and eating the feathers. Whatever supplies this want will relieve the expression of it, or, in other words, cure the habit. To this end the birds should have good feed, and a grass run if possible. If not, fine grass should be chopped up and given them, as also green food. *Bones* should be burned in the fire then pounded small, and put within their reach. This will supply the carbonate of lime, should that be wanting, and an occasional feed of wet up bran will supply the silex, should the desire arise from deprivation of that. Some animal food, well peppered, may also be used advantageously. Give also the SPECIFIC J J, morning and night. These hints and measures will be sufficient to ensure the breeder or fancier against loss from this source.

Fractures.

Broken wings or legs in fowls may be set without much trouble, if the fractured ends of bones are brought together and secured. The leg or thigh may be held straight with the broken ends neatly in position, and a rag, or even paper wet in white of egg, carefully wrapped around it several times. The white of egg hardens as it dries, and furnishes a sufficient protection until the callus is formed. Broken wings are best secured by tying the feathers firmly together about an inch from the end, after having put the fractured ends neatly in place.

Frost Bites

If the comb or wattles are frost bitten they should be at first rubbed with snow or icy cold water, until the natural color and suppleness is restored and then an application of the WITCH HAZEL OIL, or if you have not that, the MARVEL OF HEALING in fluid will do. Two or three applications of either will suffice, the oil being every way preferable.

Gapes, or Throat Worms.

This disease is so called from the peculiar action of the chickens who are affected with it. It is caused by the presence of a pale reddish worm, some three-quarters of an inch in length, which infests the mouth and throat, and of which from two to a dozen are found in a chicken, each usually doubled up. These worms are a species of *ascarus* or pin worms and have been bred like other *ascarus and strongylas* in damp earth, and hence are found among chickens which are bred in damp moist soils, and are rarely ever known when the birds have a clean, high or gravelly yard. The spawn of these worms are deposited by myriads in the moist unclean soil, and thence transplanted to the crop with the feed become developed in the throat of the chick. This is the most recent position of scientific knowledge on this subject.

The best method of cure is to remove, where possible, the chickens to a dryer locality, and to give them the SPECIFIC FOR WORMS D D, morning and night. To remove the worms from the throat, make a loop of one or two horse hairs, which thrust down the throat, and with a slight twist draw it out, bringing the worms with it. This may be repeated until the throat is cleared, or a quill feather, stripped to within an inch or two of its end, may be dipped in a mixture of glycerine or oil, and petroleum, made in the proportion of three parts of oil or glycerine to one part of petroleum Dip the feather in the mixture, and in like manner pass it into and well down the throat, and with a twist bring it out with the worms adhering. The used feathers and remaining oil should be burned to destroy the larvae of the worms, and fresh feathers used freely, so as not to spread the worms or their larvae. The ends of the fingers dipped in petroleum and applied to the body along under the wings of brooding hens, where chickens are affected, will drive off the lice, and also aid in exterminating the gapes in the chickens. It should be applied once in four or six days.

Gout or Rheumatism

May be distinguished by the birds being lame walking with difficulty, and sitting about, and on examination the legs or thighs will be found hot and feverish; or in cases of longer standing there will be evident stiffness of the joints and weakness of the legs, and in some cases contraction of the toes, which indicate cramps. The bird should be kept in a comfortable dry place, and the SPECIFIC B B, given it three times a day. It is produced by exposure to cold and wet, or to sudden change of temperature.

Leg Weakness.

In large breeds of fowls, and especially when being bred "in and in," so that the stamina of the system is lowered there is a difficient growth of bony matter, and the birds are weak, squatting around or walking on their hocks. It may be remedied by giving the SPECIFIC J J, morning and night, and bones or oyster shells should be burned in the fire, and then pounded small, and the dust occasionally mixed with the food or placed where the fowls have access to it. This will increase the deposit of ossific matter and impart strength to the legs.

Giddiness,

Which is liable to occur in over fed birds, if suffered to continue may result in apoplexy. A dose or two of the SPECIFIC A A, will equalize the circulation and remove the difficulty and danger.

Lice.

This is liable to be a terrible pest when large flocks are overcrowded, or have insufficient space, unless extra care is taken in cleanliness and thorough ventilation. The entire quarters, henhouse, roosts, and yard fences should be thoroughly cleaned and whitewashed, and all the waste straw, chaff, and manure removed, two or three times per season, certainly spring and fall After having removed and burned the waste straw and litter, the henhouse and roost should be thoroughly fumigated with sulphur. In order to do this effectually after cleaning out all the rubbish, take an old iron pot or other suitable iron or earthen vessel, and place in the bottom of it a half pound or pound of *sulphur*, either powdered or roll, and on this lay a red hot iron. After having placed it in the position best calculated to fumigate the building or roost, and close the doors and openings as far as possible. Be careful not to inhale the fumes yourself, and see that no poor chicken or other animal, is inclosed so as to be suffocated, the lice being the only objects intended for the fumigation. This being done, and a new coat of whitewash, covering everything, and fresh straw or hay for the nests, will make all sweet and wholesome again. When sifted coal ashes, or wood ashes, can be had and mixed with the sand, in which the birds wallow, lice will not trouble them, and the more so if some *flour of sulphur* is occasionally thrown into the mass. For an individual bird troubled with these vermin, a little petroleum applied along under the wings once a week will remove the pests.

Indigestion—Loss of Appetite.

If, as sometimes happens in consequence of overfeeding, or the use of too highly seasoned food, fowls loose their appetite, and the digestion and thrift is impaired a change to soft, well cooked food, and the use, night and morning, of the SPECIFIC J J, will soon correct the difficulty.

Liver Disease.

This is a more formidable complaint, mostly observed in cold damp localities, and rarely when the surroundings are dry and pure. Artificial enlargement of the liver is produced in geese by confining them in dark cellars; and fowls that have indigestion from overfeeding in similar conditions, will have liver disease with enlargement of that organ, a dull, stupid appearance and a yellowish tint about the head and comb. It may be cured by giving the SPECIFIC J J, morning and night, or in obstinate cases giving the SPECIFIC C C, in like manner. The bird should have soft or cooked food and a dry situation.

Moulting.

We should take into consideration the great drain upon the system of fowls in Moulting. Not only are the ordinary wastes of the body to be maintained, but the old summer coat of feathers is to be discarded and an entirely new one to be produced involving in its growth all the essential elements of which the feathers are composed. If these substances —lime, carbon, sulphur, silex, etc., are not to be had in the food provided for them or are imperfectly produced or eliminated, the work drags and the organism suffers, and waste of flesh, poverty of the system, or illness is the result Hence it is a wise precaution, during the season of Moulting, to allow the flock a more generous supply of food, and of better quality than usual, and to exercise more than ordinary care in housing and shelter. Fowls that have fair feed and a reasonable range will rarely require special care, but those confined are more apt to suffer. Any stimulating food is of advantage. Hemp seed is very beneficial, and iron is invaluable. An *acetate* of *iron* may be readily made by putting some nails or other bits of iron in *cider*. This, after standing a day or two, may be used in mixing the feed. More cider may be added as required, and so the cider and iron may be kept and used during the entire Moulting season. The SPECIFIC J J, is the proper remedy, and should also be given two or three times per week, or even more frequently if the birds are suffering much.

A little care and attention in this respect will shorten the period of Moulting, and bring the birds out in better health and vigor and better plumage.

Pip or Chirp.

Young chickens are affected by a peculiar form of disease termed Pip or Chirp, from the short spasmodic chirups which they make during the complaint. The chickens mope about uttering this peculiar cry, and seek refuge in solitary places, as it is the instinct of animals and birds to pick at, maim or destroy the sick or maimed among them. The chicken is hot and feverish although trembling violently, and they are extremely tender on being handled, and soon a dark colored, dry horny scale will be found at the end of the tongue, and the beak may turn yellow at the base; the appetite fails and the plumage becomes ruffled, and they gradually sink and die. It is doubtless caused by exposure to wet weather, as the light down is easily saturated, and is long in drying. The SPECIFIC A A, may be given at first, one or two doses, and afterwards the SPECIFIC J J, three times per day. The removal of the scale at the end of the tongue is of no consequence. That is not the cause of the disease but the result, and the tongue will come all right so soon as the chick is restored in his circulation and digestion. Of course the birds should be well housed and fed on soft food.

Roup.

Almost all forms of chronic catarrh in fowls go by the name of Roup. It usually begins as a severe cold, caused by exposure to cold, wet and damp. There is discharge from the nostrils, at first of thin mucus, and which soon becomes opaque and even offensive, and the entire cavity of the nose may become filled up; froth and mucus fill the inner angle of the eye, the lids are swelled and often the eye ball quite concealed, and in severe cases the entire face is considerably swelled. It is said to be contagious, but is probably only so in extremely virulent cases. But the fact that a flock of fowls are exposed to similar disease making conditions, and that many are taken nearly at the same time, would countenance the idea of its contagious character. The causes of the disease should be avoided by providing shelter for chickens during the cold, chilly fall nights, and not permitting them to wander around without feed in the cold raw mornings. A plentiful supply of nourishing food and comfortable shelter when sudden cold changes of weather occur, will do much to prevent the appearance of this disease, and the consequent loss. The iron and cider with the food will be useful, and onions cut up fine and mixed in the soft feed, is also an invaluable agent for fowls affected with any form of Roup. The SPECIFIC A A, is the proper remedy, two or three doses at first during the inflammatory stage. Then the SPECIFIC C C for CATARRH and INFLUENZA is the proper remedy, and may be relied upon for a cure. Give it as often as three, or even four times, per day, in extreme cases. Of course the severe cases should be well housed, have warm and dry lodgings, free from exposure of open windows and cold drafts of air, as the bird is liable to new chill from fresh exposure. Washing the head and syringing out the nose, and washing the throat with salt and vinegar, or even with water and castile soap, is rarely necessary and really of very little consequence. As the catarrh passes off the secretions will become healthy and natural, and all these discharges disappear.

Rump-Ail, or Wry Tail.

These are conditions arising from faulty organization or insufficient keep, and have for symptoms constipation, drooping head, ruffled feathers, or the tail carried to one side. In some cases a swelling appears upon the rump which may suppurate and form an abscess, which had better be opened if matter has formed. The SPECIFIC J J is the proper remedy, and may be given two or three times per day. Where such conditions appear at all frequently in a breed of fowls, it indicates an inherent weakness, and the breed had better be changed or crossed with more vigorous stock.

Soft Eggs

May be a sign of over-feeding, but is more commonly from the want of material of which to form the shell—lime, starch, sulphur, etc. The flock should have an occasional feed of mashed potatoes and lime, old mortar, burnt oyster shells, pounded up, should be placed in reach. An occasional dose of SPECIFIC J J will be beneficial.

INDEX.

PAGE.

Published by

Facsimile Publisher
Ashok Vihar, Delhi-110052 (India)
Website: www.facsimilepublishers.com

Distributed by

Gyan Books Pvt. Ltd.
5, Ansari Road, Daryaganj, New Delhi-110002 (India)
E-mail: books@gyanbooks.com, Website: www.gyanbooks.com

9 789333 166010